Workbook to Accompany
Fundamentals of Emergency Care

Dedication

For Bob, whose belief in me is neverending.
To Genna and Kim, firefighters after their father, EMTs after their mother,
unique individuals in their own right.

Acknowledgments

I would like to extend a special thanks to Howard Huth III, NREMT-P,
paramedic in the town of Guilderland, for his help with editing the workbook.

Workbook to Accompany
Fundamentals of Emergency Care

Richard W. O. Beebe, MEd, RN, NREMT-P
Program Director
Bassett Healthcare
Center for Rural Emergency Medical Services Education
Cooperstown, New York

Adjunct Faculty
Herkimer County Community College
Herkimer, New York

Deborah L. Funk, MD, NREMT-P
Instructor
Emergency Medicine
Albany Medical College
Albany, New York

Attending Physician
Emergency Department
Albany Medical Center Hospital
Albany, New York

Workbook written by:
Deborah Kufs, BS, RN, CCRN, CEN, NREMT-P
Clinical Instructor
Institute for Prehospital Emergency Medicine
Hudson Valley Community College
Troy, New York

DELMAR

THOMSON LEARNING ™   Australia Canada Mexico Singapore Spain United Kingdom United States

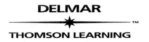

DELMAR
THOMSON LEARNING™

Workbook to Accompany
Fundamentals of Emergency Care
Richard W. O. Beebe and Deborah L. Funk

Workbook written by: Deborah Kufs, BS, RN, NREMT-P

Business Unit Director:
William Brottmiller

Channel Manager:
Tara Carter

Executive Editor:
Cathy L. Esperti

Project Editor:
Maureen M. E. Grealish

Developmental Editor:
Darcy M. Scelsi

Production Coordinator:
John Mickelbank

Editorial Assistant:
Jill Korznat

Production Editor:
Mary Colleen Liburdi

Executive Marketing Manager:
Dawn F. Gerrain

For permission to use material from this text or product, contact us by
Tel   (800) 730-2214
Fax   (800) 730-2215
www.thomsonrights.com

Library of Congress Catalog Card Number: 00-050889
ISBN: 0-7668-1493-9

CONTENTS

Section Six: Emergency Medical Care

Section Seven: Trauma Care

Section Eight: Maternal Health Emergencies

Section Nine: Childhood Emergencies

Section Ten: Geriatric Care

Section Eleven: EMS Operations

PREFACE

This workbook was designed to accompany *Fundamentals of Emergency Care*. It is part of a complete system, including the main text, an instructor's manual, a test bank, an image library, a PowerPoint presentation and a Web tutor.

The workbook includes exercises designed to help the student review text material, key terms, and skills. It provides step-by-step progression from understanding terminology to learning discrete skills and concepts to applying the material.

Prehospital emergency care is a combination of thinking and doing. The workbook material challenges the student to acquire the basic knowledge, use critical thinking skills, and develop the hands-on skills necessary for practice as an EMT-Basic.

Regulations covering the practice of prehospital emergency care vary from state to state; therefore, it is important for the student to learn the specific regulation in his area.

CHAPTER 1 INTRODUCTION TO EMERGENCY MEDICAL SERVICES

EMTs are the foundation of the prehospital component of Emergency Medical Services. This review will assist you in recalling historical events and reflecting upon their implications for your new vocation.

Matching: Match the following with their descriptions:

1. _____ Certified First Responders

2. _____ EMT-Basic

3. _____ EMT-Intermediate

4. _____ EMT-Paramedic

5. _____ EMD

6. _____ Good Samaritan

7. _____ NHTSA

8. _____ Star of Life

9. _____ Emergency Physician

10. _____ white paper

a. national EMS symbol

b. laid groundwork for inclusion of EMS in federal legislation

c. a national level of care that involves administering oxygen and simple bleeding control

d. a doctor trained to give care to the acutely ill or injured

e. one who would stop and help

f. a method of questioning callers and giving life-saving instructions

g. most common prehospital provider

h. a branch of the Department of Transportation

i. highest level of prehospital care provider

j. provider trained in advanced airway management and IV therapy

True or False: Read each statement and decide if it is TRUE or FALSE. Place T or F on line before each statement.

1. _____ Providing care to the sick or injured can be traced back to ancient times.

2. _____ Modern Emergency Medical Service is designed only for lifesaving care.

3. _____ The military had little involvement in the development of modern EMS.

4. _____ The American Red Cross was formed by Deke Farrington.

5. _____ The "White Paper" was written to describe death in the Vietnam War.

6. _____ OSHA was formed to meet the needs of EMTs, and to speak to the public about EMS.

7. _____ Universal Access is designed so that all emergency services can be reached by a 3-digit number.

8. _____ Emergency Medical Dispatch consists of lifesaving phone instructions and triage.

9. _____ EMT-Bs work only on ambulances.

10. _____ Paramedics are the highest trained prehospital care providers.

Short Answer: Read each question. Think about the information presented in your text, and then answer each question with one or two sentences.

1. The concept of the "ambulances volante" is still practiced today. From the text, give an example.

2. Why did soldiers in Vietnam have a greater chance for survival than drivers and pedestrians in the United States?

3. Johnny and Roy led the American public to think differently about people suffering illnesses or injuries before they could get to a hospital. What did this change in thinking do for health care?

4. What components are necessary for a successful "EMS Chain of Survival"?

5. Which of these components is influenced by the EMT-B?

6. How is EMS provided in your community?

7. What changes do you expect to see in the future of EMS?

8. How do the various prehospital care providers, communicators, physicians, and allied health professionals contribute to the concepts drawn from the "Star of Life"?

CHAPTER 2 MEDICAL RESPONSIBILITIES

The EMT-B provides medical care to patients in many different settings. Responsibility for safety, quality care, and adhering to standards belongs to the EMT-B when providing medical care.

Ordering: Place the following duties in the order in which they should be performed for a call. Put a numeral 1 before the first duty, a 2 before the next, and so on.

_____ Assess patient

_____ Call medical control as needed

_____ Continue care during transport

_____ Determine mechanism of injury or nature of illness

_____ Drive safely to scene

_____ Give verbal and written reports to staff

_____ Replace any equipment used

_____ Move patient to the ambulance

_____ Notify destination facility of patient

_____ Perform scene size-up

_____ Reassess patient

_____ Receive information from dispatch

Identification: Place an X in front of those patient-care responsibilities performed by EMT-Bs.

_____ Airway maintenance   _____ Hemorrhage control

_____ Ventilation of patients   _____ Suturing of wounds

_____ Intubation of patients   _____ Bandaging of wounds

_____ CPR   _____ Assisting in childbirth

_____ Defibrillation by AED   _____ Prescribing medications to patients

_____ Manual cardioversion

True or False: Read each statement and decide if it is TRUE or FALSE. Place T or F on line before each statement.

1. _____ The first priority of any EMT-B is personal safety.

2. _____ Good safety precautions always involve complicated procedures.

3. _____ EMT-Bs should never remove a patient from a dangerous situation until medical care has been provided.

4. _____ Continuing medical education is necessary for EMT-Bs.

5. _____ After the EMT-B takes a state written exam, he will be licensed to practice in that state.

6. _____ Quality management is an administrative role performed by the agency's top administrative officer.

7. _____ Retrospective quality assessment is performed by a team member accompanying the crews on calls.

Definitions: Write the definitions of the following terms.

1. certification   _____

2. medical direction   _____

3. off-line medical control   _____

4. on-line medical control   _____

5. quality management   _____

6. professional conduct   _____

8. quality improvement   _____

9. prehospital health care team _____

Identification: Read each of the following statements and determine if it describes classroom (didactic), hands-on (psychomotor), or clinical (integration) opportunity. Place the correct word on the line in front of the statement.

1. _____ The instructor assigns readings from the text.

2. _____ The student completes medical rounds with an Emergency Physician.

3. _____ A student is moulaged (made up), while another assesses for injuries.

4. _____ A case study is presented, and the class describes care.

5. _____ A student observes and plans care while riding with an EMT-B on an ambulance.

Short Answer: Read each question. Think about the information presented in your text, and then answer each question with one or two sentences.

1. Why is it important for the EMT to reassure bystanders during a call?

2. Explain the value of a clean identifiable uniform and nametag.

3. Why must the EMT-B consider added training after his initial course?

Critical Thinking 1: Read the following case study and answer the questions after it.

Jenna, Kimberley, and Andy were called to the home of an older female patient who had difficulty breathing. After the call was completed and the ambulance restocked, they stopped for a well-deserved meal at the local diner. The EMTs were annoyed that a woman would continue to smoke, even after her doctor had advised her not to do so. They talked amongst themselves about the patient, her obvious lack of commitment to taking care of herself, and their resentment at being called frequently just "because she won't listen to her doctor."

1. Based on the EMT Code of Ethics, what did the EMTs in this study violate?

2. How would you feel if the patient in this scenario were your relative?

3. Based on the Code of Ethics, what actions could the EMTs take in promoting a healthier lifestyle choice?

Critical Thinking 2: Read the following case study and answer the questions after it.

The captain of the ambulance squad was frustrated. Four times in the last month, patients were dropped off at the hospital without immobilization of swollen, deformed, painful extremities. Nothing in the run reports indicated that a more pressing need was assigned priority, and to make things worse, nothing even indicated that the injuries were found and assessed! Something had to change!

1. What five elements must be performed to ensure the ultimate goal of quality medical care?

2. What two forms of assessment are available to team members in evaluating the care that was given?

3. Which of these has the captain of the ambulance squad used?

4. Based on Quality Management elements, suggest a way in which the captain can help promote improvements in care for patients with injured extremities.

Critical Thinking 3: Read the following case study and answer the questions after it.

Bonnie and Howard answered a call for a man who had been stung by a bee. When they arrived, he told them that he had been stung several times while in his backyard and was now having some trouble breathing. He said that he had a history of allergy to stings, had an epi-pen prescribed, but that it was in his coat pocket and he couldn't get to it. Howard obtained the epi-pen as Bonnie completed an initial assessment, and got a set of vital signs. Based on the procedures in their community, they assisted the man in self-injecting the medication. They continued with oxygen administration and transported the man to the hospital for evaluation. During transport, they reassessed him, and Howard spoke with the physician at the receiving hospital. He received orders to administer oxygen by a different device. The patient was dropped off at the hospital. A week after this call, the agency's medical director reviewed the call with Howard and Bonnie, complimenting them on a job well done, and making a suggestion for improvement in the future.

1. Which actions are based on off-line medical control?

2. Which are based on on-line medical control?

3. In what way did Howard and Bonnie act as the physician's designated agent?

CHAPTER 3 THE LEGAL RESPONSIBILITIES OF THE EMT

Emergency medical service is considered a public trust. The public expects prompt, professional care plus attention to individual rights.

Completion: Complete the missing word in each sentence.

1. A _ _ _ _ _ _ _ _ _ _ t is leaving unsupervised a patient who is in your care.

2. A breach of _ _ _ fi _ _ _ _ _ _ _ _ _ _ _ _ occurs when a person divulges information about another without permission.

3. An awareness of the importance of preserving evidence at the scene of a crime constitutes e _ _ _ e _ _ _ _ _ o _ _ _ _ _ _ _.

4. _ _ _ _ S _ _ _ _ _ _ _ _ n _ _ _ s were designed to protect certain classes of people when they are helping others.

5. H _ _ _ _ _ C _ _ _ P _ _ _ _ enables a person to make care decisions for someone who is not capable of doing so.

6. A presumption that a person would agree to be treated if he could agree defines i _ _ _ _ _ _ c _ _ _ _ _ _ _.

7. A person who is required by law to take a particular action has a l _ _ _ _ d _ _ _ to _ _ _.

8. Written instructions for an EMT is part of _ _ _-_ _ _ _ medical control.

9. Speaking with the doctor on the radio is part of _ _-_ _ _ _ medical control.

10. The patient's _ _ _ _ of _ _ _ _ _ _ _ are what the patient expects when being cared for in a hospital or health facility.

11. A group of injuries common to a certain mechanism is called a p _ _ _ _ _ _ of _ _ _ _ _ _.

12. Restriction of a patient's freedom by ties or cravats is called physical _ _ _ _ _ _ _ _ _ _.

13. An action or inaction that is the direct reason for harm is termed c _ _ _ _ _ _ _ _ of i _ _ _ _ _.

14. The level of care recognized as being required is a _ _ _ _ _ _ _ _ of care.

Identification: Read the following and determine the type of consent in each case. Write the type on the line in front of the case.

1. _____ When the EMT tells Mrs. Jones that he needs to obtain a blood pressure reading, she rolls up her sleeve and holds out her arm.

2. _____ The school nurse gives permission for the EMT to examine a child injured on the playground.

3. _____ The EMTs assess a man who is unconscious. He is at the mall and no one is with him.

4. _____ The police ask the EMT to assess a severely injured man they are arresting.

5. _____ The EMTs provide care to a child who is choking and cannot breathe.

6. _____ Mr. Jones tells the EMTs that he called 911 because he couldn't breathe well.

7. _____ Mrs. Brown gives permission for the EMT to bandage a cut on her 3-year-old daughter's arm.

8. _____ While home from the Army, 17-year-old Jeff gives permission for the EMT to assess him after a motor vehicle collision.

True or False: Read each statement and decide if it is TRUE or FALSE. Place T or F on line before each statement.

1. _____ Apnea (not breathing) is considered a sign of irreversible death.

2. _____ Lividity can be reversed with adequate oxygenation.

3. _____ Decapitation is defined as severing of the head from the body.

4. _____ A mortal wound means the patient can survive his injuries with routine care.

5. _____ A DNR means that the EMT cannot treat the patient without a direct physician's order.

6. _____ A living will expresses the patient's wishes in regard to prolonging life.

7. _____ EMTs are not involved in the care of patients dying from a terminal illness.

8. _____ Stiffening of the muscles after death is called decomposition.

Identification: Circle the five elements in a malpractice case that must be proved for the EMT to be liable for negligence.

standard of care   a criminal action

protocols   allegations

duty to act   harm

a mistake   causation of injury

a failure to meet standards

Yes or No: Read each of the following statements and decide if the EMTs can disclose the patient information or not. Write YES if they can, or NO if they cannot do so legally.

1. _____ A police officer asks if the patient admitted to smoking marijuana.

2. _____ A doctor who is a friend of the patient's father asks what the patient's chief complaint is.

3. _____ An emergency department nurse asks for the patient's vital signs.

4. _____ Witnesses to an accident ask if the patient is the school superintendent.

5. _____ An insurance adjuster asks the EMTs if the accident was caused by the patient.

6. _____ A surgeon called by the Emergency Physician asks about the patient's position in the vehicle.

7. _____ The patient's mother asks if her daughter admitted to being pregnant.

8. _____ A lawyer asks to read the patient care report.

9. _____ A nurse at the hospital asks if you transported her friend to the emergency department.

10. _____ The physician's assistant asks for a list of the patient's medications for the emergency department chart.

Identification: Place an X in front of the appropriate behaviors when dealing with a crime scene.

_____ Keep unnecessary people off the scene

_____ Use the patient's telephone to avoid radio communications

_____ Leave all medical materials on scene

_____ Turn off lights

_____ Remember anything that must be moved for patient care

_____ Do not touch weapons

_____ Leave answering machines or caller identification devices alone

_____ Cover the body to maintain modesty

_____ Do not use sink to wash hands

_____ Turn off TV, radio, and video equipment

Short Answer: Read each question. Think about the information presented in your text, and then answer each question with one or two sentences.

1. What conditions must be identified before a patient can be allowed to refuse medical assistance?

2. Explain the value of good listening skills when a patient is refusing medical care or assistance.

Critical Thinking 1: Read the following case study and answer the questions after it.

Sixteen-year-old Amy and her boyfriend, Aaron, have had sexual relations on several occasions. Amy has been feeling sick lately and is concerned that she may be pregnant or have developed symptoms of a disease. At her clinic visit, Amy signs her own consent form.

1. Why can the clinic accept Amy's consent for assessment and treatment?

2. List other circumstances in which an EMT could accept consent from a minor.

Critical Thinking 2: Read the following case study and answer the questions after it.

Brenda and Jeff have been dispatched to a home for a 60-year-old man who is having chest pressure. The man, Mr. Rotelli, appears ill as they enter the residence. His wife has called EMS even though the patient is saying that this is the result of too much sausage and peppers the night before. Mr. Rotelli tells the EMTs that he doesn't need to go to the hospital.

1. What should the EMTs say to Mr. Rotelli?

2. If Mr. Rotelli still doesn't want to go to the hospital, what should they do next?

3. What must be documented regarding Mr. Rotelli's refusal?

Critical Thinking 3: Read the following case study and answer the question after it.

Andrew and Dory are called to the home of a 65-year-old female patient who has a history of breast cancer. Mr. Johnson called EMS because his wife was in pain. When the EMTs arrive, they find Mrs. Johnson slumped over on the couch. Initial assessment shows her not to be breathing and without a pulse. As Dory prepares to begin CPR, Andrew says he would grab the defibrillator. Mr. Johnson tells them to please stop as his wife doesn't want anything like that. She has a DNR order, but he doesn't know where it is.

1. What should Dory and Andrew do next?

Critical Thinking 4: Read the following case study and answer the questions after it.

Kandy and Tom arrive on the scene of a 5-year-old boy who has a leg injury. The little boy won't talk to them, or to his parents who tell the EMTs that their son fell off the swing set several hours ago. The little boy, Jason, ignores the EMTs as they attempt to assess his leg and find out where it hurts. His parents then tell the EMTs that Jason knew he shouldn't have been on the slide and that they knew he would hurt himself someday.

1. What should the EMTs observe about the parents and child?

2. What should Kandy and Tom report to the Emergency Department staff?

CHAPTER 4 STRESS IN EMERGENCY MEDICAL SERVICES

The EMT-B will be faced with many emotional and stressful situations. These situations can cause physical and emotional reactions. The EMT-B must recognize the common stressors and plan to handle them effectively.

Completion: Complete each line by choosing the correct word or phrase from the Key Terms found in Chapter 4 of the textbook.

_ _ _ _ **S** _ _ _ _ _ _ _ _ isolation

_ _ _ **T** _ stress

_ _ **R** _ _ _ _

_ **E** _ _ _ _ _ _ _ _

healthy _ _ _ _ **S** _ _ _ _

scene **S** _ _ _ _ _ _

_ _ **R** _ _ _ _ _ _

relaxation **E** _ _ _ _ _ _ _ _

multiple _ _ **S** _ _ _ _ _ incident

_ _ _ _ _ _ _ or _ _ _ _ _ _ _ _ _ **P** _ _ _ _

_ _ _ _ **O** _ _ _ _ stress

_ **N** _ _ _ _ time

_ _ _ _ _ **S**

diversionary _ _ _ _ _ _ _ _ _ _ **E** _

Matching: Place the letter of the correct definition on the line in front of the term.

1. _____ stress

2. _____ stressor

3. _____ fight or flight response

4. _____ unwind time

5. _____ healthy lifestyle

6. _____ burnout

7. _____ debriefing

8. _____ CISM team

9. _____ acute stress

10. _____ chronic stress

a. a single event that causes a stress reaction

b. physical, emotional, behavioral response of the body to changing conditions

c. exercise, balanced diet, no smoking

d. events that trigger stress

e. team discussion of details of an event

f. opportunity to relax

g. repeated events affecting the EMT over time

h. specially trained people whose job it is to prevent negative impact of events

i. condition that arises from chronic stress

j. response of the body to stress by preparing to run or defend itself

Sorting: Read each of the following and determine if it describes physical, emotional, or behavioral signs of chronic stress exposure. Place the word or phrase under the correct category.

alcohol abuse   gastrointestinal distress

aggression   headaches

anger   increased heart rate

anxiety   insomnia

avoidance   irritability

depression   muscle tension

drug abuse   procrastination

edgy   withdrawal

fatigue

Physical   **Emotional**   **Behavioral**

Short Answer: Read each question. Think about the information presented in your text, and then answer each question with one or two sentences.

1. Why would prevention of stressful situations be preferable to treating stress reactions?

2. List two ways in which EMTs can decrease the number of encounters with high stress situations?

Critical Thinking 1: Read each of the following and think of a way that the perception can be changed. Write your answer below.

1. Jaime is angry because the nurse in the ED didn't answer her question.

2. Ginny is scared to begin her new job as an EMT-B.

3. Patrick can't sleep after a call in which a man with cancer died in the ambulance.

4. Greg develops a queasy feeling whenever he brings a patient to the cardiac cath lab.

Critical Thinking 2: Read the following case study and answer the questions after it.

Liz had been practicing as an EMT for several years when she decided to return to school and become a paramedic. It was hard work, but her colleagues supported her efforts. Today was the big day; she expected her test results in the mail. As expected, she scored well and would be on her way to different responsibilities. Her coworkers were cheering when Liz broke down in tears and said she had no interest in being a paramedic.

1. Could Liz be experiencing stress? Why or why not?

2. How could Liz alter the perception of this event?

Critical Thinking 3: Read the following case study and answer the questions after it.

Geoff had finally finished a long shift. There were many calls in the previous 24 hours and most had involved both physical care of the patient, and much explanation to each family. One gentleman had suffered from chest pain, and his family had difficulty understanding the need for an oxygen mask. A young child had been found lethargic and ill this morning, and the doctors think she may have meningitis. Geoff may even need some medications to prevent him from developing the illness. Two youngsters were playing by the road and one suffered an arm injury after being hit by a car. The shift went on and on. When Geoff arrived home, he discovered that his wife had given their 4-year-old son some medication for a fever. Geoff became very angry and upset. He started yelling at his wife and even screamed at the dog.

1. From the case study, list at least five events that may be stressful for Geoff.

2. List five diversionary techniques that may help Geoff manage stress.

Critical Thinking 4: Read the following case study and answer the questions after it.

Mr. Linkowski was being transported to the dialysis facility for the third treatment this week. He was very quiet, but did mention that he wouldn't be seeing the crew next week as he knew that he would not live through the weekend. Janice, the EMT, tried to cheer him up, but only succeeded in making herself feel worse. Back at the station, she complained of feeling sick to her stomach and having a headache.

1. What is the likely cause of Janice's illness?

2. Suggest a reason for this to occur.

3. How can Janice change her perception of this event?

Critical Thinking 5: Read the following case study and answer the questions after it.

The Midtown Ambulance Service was dispatched to a motor vehicle collision in front of the high school. The media was already there. The collision was relatively minor, didn't involve any of the school kids, and could be handled by only one ambulance crew. Joe, an EMT who had participated in a much more severe call in front of the high school in his hometown, kept yelling that they should get more ambulances ready and get the cameras out of his way.

1. What is the likely cause of Joe's reaction?

2. What are some of the signs that Joe's crew members should be aware of regarding Joe's behavior?

CHAPTER 5 ANATOMY AND PHYSIOLOGY

In order to understand a patient's illness or injury, the EMT-B must have a basic understanding of human anatomy and physiology.

Matching: Match word or words with its definition.

1. _____ anatomy
2. _____ physiology
3. _____ standard anatomic position
4. _____ medial
5. _____ lateral
6. _____ superior
7. _____ inferior
8. _____ distal
9. _____ proximal
10. _____ bilateral
11. _____ superficial
12. _____ dorsal
13. _____ apex
14. _____ base
15. _____ inversion
16. _____ eversion
17. _____ prone
18. _____ supine
19. _____ Fowler's position
20. _____ unilateral
21. _____ recovery position
22. _____ abduction
23. _____ adduction
24. _____ extension
25. _____ flexion

a. outward movement, as in a foot twisting out
b. to move away from the body
c. movement of a joint that narrows the angle
d. directional term for both sides of the body
e. lying face down
f. turning inward
g. a reference, facing forward, palms forward
h. top of an object
i. sitting at a 45–60 degree angle
j. lying face up
k. study of the structure of an organism
l. side of a structure
m. study of function of an organism
n. away from core of the body
o. at or near the surface
p. also known as left lateral recovery position
q. a point on one side of the body
r. toward the core of the trunk of the body
s. lower than the reference point
t. movement of a joint that widens the angle
u. bottom of an object
v. to move toward the body
w. toward midline of the body
x. back of a surface
y. point of a triangle

Integumentary System

Fill in the Blank:

1. One of the most important functions of the skin is that it _____ us from disease.

2. The _____ is the outermost layer of the skin.

3. Capillaries and nerve endings are found in the _____.

4. Fat stored within the _____ layer serves as insulation.

5. The _____ of the skin serves as a diagnostic tool.

Muscular System

True or False: Read each statement and decide if it is TRUE or FALSE. Place T or F on the line before each statement.

1. _____ The ability of muscles to shorten permits movement.

2. _____ The temporal muscle is considered an accessory breathing muscle.

3. _____ The biceps, triceps, and deltoid muscles are located in the lower arm.

4. _____ The thoracic muscle divides the abdominal cavity from the chest cavity.

5. _____ The quadriceps permits extension of the leg.

Skeletal System

Matching: Match each area with its correct description by placing the letter on the line.

1. _____ appendicular skeleton
2. _____ axial skeleton
3. _____ foot
4. _____ hand
5. _____ lower arm
6. _____ lower leg
7. _____ patella
8. _____ pelvic girdle
9. _____ shoulder girdle
10. _____ skull
11. _____ spinal column
12. _____ sternum
13. _____ thoracic cage
14. _____ upper arm
15. _____ upper leg

a. includes skull, ribs, and spinal column

b. has multiple facial bones and the cranium

c. has a series of bones stacked on top of each other

d. surrounds and protects the heart and lungs

e. also called the breastbone

f. description of the bones forming the limbs

g. made up of the clavicle and the scapulas

h. the humerus

i. also called the forearm

j. carpals, metacarpals, and phalanges

k. supports all the weight of the body

l. has the longest and strongest bone in the body

m. a bony disc that protects the inner joint

n. contains the tibia and the fibula

o. contains the tarsals and calcaneus

Labeling: Label each diagram in Figure 5–1 with the names of the bones shown.

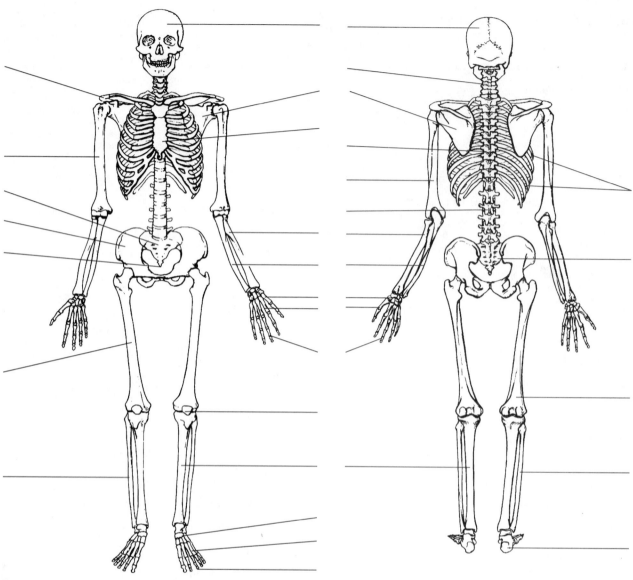

Figure 5–1

Central Nervous System

Fill in the Blank:

The central nervous system is made up of the _____ and the _____ _____. It is involved in the _____ and _____ of all control messages in the body. The brain consists of the _____, the _____, and the _____ _____. The brain stem consists of the _____, _____, and _____. The brain stem controls life sustaining functions such as _____ and _____. The "athletic brain" is called the _____. The "athletic brain" controls _____ _____. The largest area of the brain, the seat of higher thinking, is called the _____. The brain is protected by three membranes called the _____ _____, _____, and the _____ _____. The brain is also protected by a fluid called _____ _____. The spinal cord begins at the _____ of the _____. The _____ _____ _____ is made up of nerves that run from the spinal cord to take messages to the body. Automatic functions such as the heart beating are under control of the _____ _____ _____.

Labeling: Label the diagram of the central nervous system in Figure 5–2.

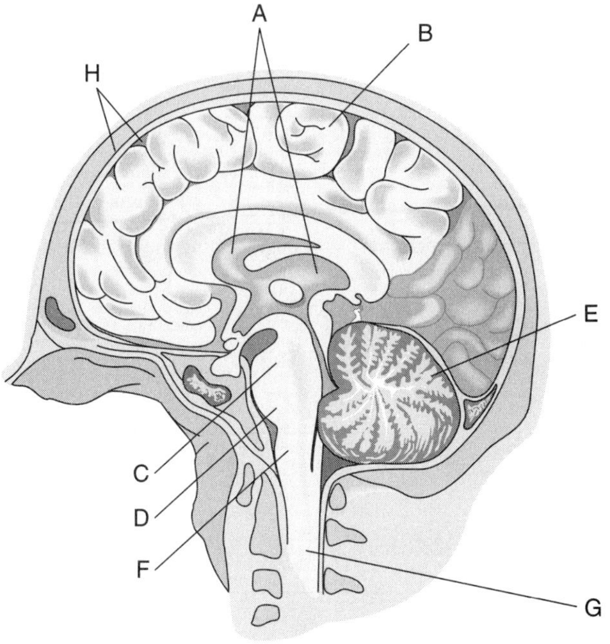

A. _____

B. _____

C. _____

D. _____

E. _____

F. _____

G. _____

H. _____

Figure 5–2

Endocrine System

Fill in the Blank:

The _____ _____ produces _____, which are chemicals designed to help the nervous system maintain control of the body. The chemicals are produced by organs called _____, and are excreted into the _____. They then affect _____ organs to change the way the organs function. The pancreas is relevant to the EMT-B because it produces _____ that helps the body use _____. Diabetics cannot produce this chemical.

Circulatory System

True or False: Read each statement and decide if it is TRUE or FALSE. Place T or F on the line before each statement.

1. _____ The action of blood flowing is called circulation.

2. _____ Blood vessels are unable to alter their size and distribution.

3. _____ The heart is located between the sternum and the spine.

4. _____ The heart is covered by a tough membrane called the arachnoid.

5. _____ The right side of the heart (right pump) sends blood to the systemic circuit.

6. _____ Each side of the heart has a receiving chamber called an atrium.

7. _____ The atria perform the actual work of circulating the blood to the tissues.

8. _____ Capillaries allow tissues to extract oxygen and nutrients from the blood.

9. _____ The largest artery in the body is called the vena cava.

10. _____ Vessels that return blood to the heart are called veins.

Fill in the Blank:

Beginning at the _____ _____, a drop of blood flows past the _____ valve and into the right _____. From there it passes the _____ valve, into the pulmonary _____, and onto the lungs. Passing through the pulmonary circulation, the drop of blood returns to the left _____ by the pulmonary _____. Moving through the left side of the heart, the blood passes the _____ valve into the left _____, passes the _____ valve and into the _____, which is the largest artery in the body. This artery helps deliver blood to body tissues. Oxygen and nutrients are removed, and the blood returns to the right atrium via the _____ _____.

Labeling: Label the diagram of the heart in Figure 5–3.

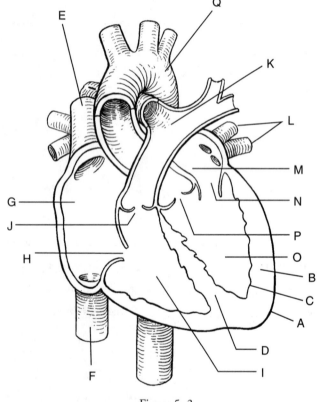

Figure 5–3

A. _____

B. _____

C. _____

D. _____

E. _____

F. _____

G. _____

H. _____

I. _____

J. _____

K. _____

L. _____

M. _____

N. _____

O. _____

P. _____

Q. _____

Respiratory System

Matching: Match word or words with its definition.

1. _____ ventilation
2. _____ respiration
3. _____ upper airway
4. _____ lower airway
5. _____ trachea
6. _____ larynx
7. _____ epiglottis
8. _____ carina
9. _____ bronchus
10. _____ alveoli
11. _____ parietal pleura
12. _____ diaphragm
13. _____ visceral pleura
14. _____ bronchioles
15. _____ oropharynx

a. air sacs that permit exchange of oxygen and CO_2
b. cartilage tubes that carry air to the lungs
c. small muscular tubes connecting to the alveoli
d. point where the right and left bronchi begin
e. muscle separating the chest from the abdomen
f. protects the trachea from foreign bodies
g. section of airway visible from the mouth
h. contains the vocal cords
i. lung covering that lines the chest wall
j. exchange of gases
k. tube that connects upper airway to lungs
l. movement of air in and out of lungs
m. lung covering that covers the lungs
n. purpose is to clean the outside air
o. includes terminal bronchioles and lungs

Labeling: Label each section of the airway on the diagram in Figure 5–4.

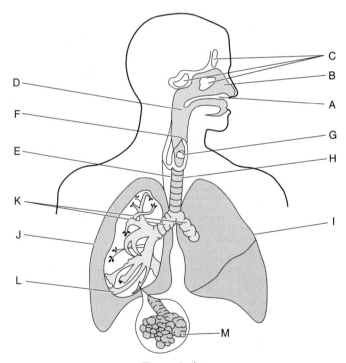

Figure 5–4

A. _____
B. _____
C. _____
D. _____
E. _____
F. _____
G. _____
H. _____
I. _____
J. _____
K. _____
L. _____
M. _____

Digestive System

Fill in the Blank: Trace the movement of food through the body by completing the following.

The beginning of digestion takes place in the _____. There, the teeth grind the food and allow it to be mixed with _____, a digestive enzyme. The mass of moistened, chewed food is called a _____ and it passes the oropharynx and into the _____, a muscular tube connected to the stomach. There, stomach _____ and other enzymes break the food apart. The stomach empties into the _____ intestine where 90% of the digestion actually takes place. This intestine takes up the largest part of the abdominal cavity. Food then moves into the _____ intestine, which terminates at the rectum. The rectum forms the feces, or waste products, which are expelled through the anus.

Completion: Complete the following table.

Organ	Type	Location	Function
liver	_____	_____	detoxifies poisons
_____	hollow	_____	stores bile
pancreas	_____	center	_____
appendix	_____	_____	unknown
_____	solid	retroperitoneal	_____

Labeling: Label the diagram of the digestive system in Figure 5–5.

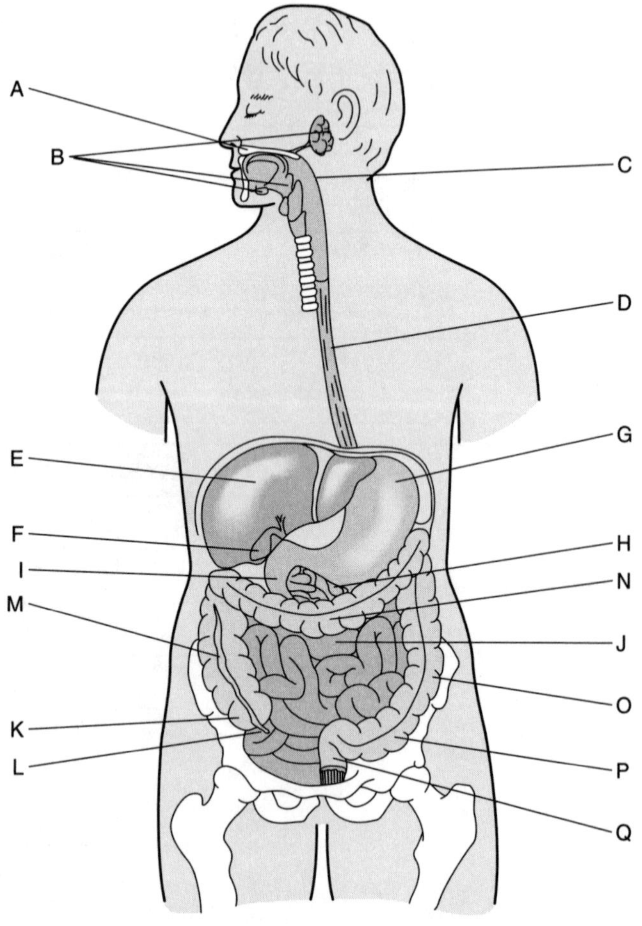

Figure 5–5

A. _____

B. _____

C. _____

D. _____

E. _____

F. _____

G. _____

H. _____

I. _____

J. _____

K. _____

L. _____

M. _____

N. _____

O. _____

P. _____

Q. _____

Reproductive System

Matching: Match word or words with its definition.

1. ____ testes
2. ____ scrotum
3. ____ penis
4. ____ sperm
5. ____ prostate
6. ____ ovary
7. ____ fallopian tube
8. ____ uterus
9. ____ menstruation
10. ____ vagina
11. ____ gonads

a. male and female organs of reproduction
b. monthly flow resulting if fertilization doesn't occur
c. produces female sex hormones
d. conduit for sperm or urine
e. gland that produces fluid to transport sperm
f. sac enclosing testes
g. responsible for fertilization of egg
h. male gonad
i. organ where a fetus grows and matures
j. allows for delivery of baby
k. allows egg to go from ovary to uterus

Labeling: Label the diagrams of the male and female reproductive systems in Figures 5–6a and 5–6b.

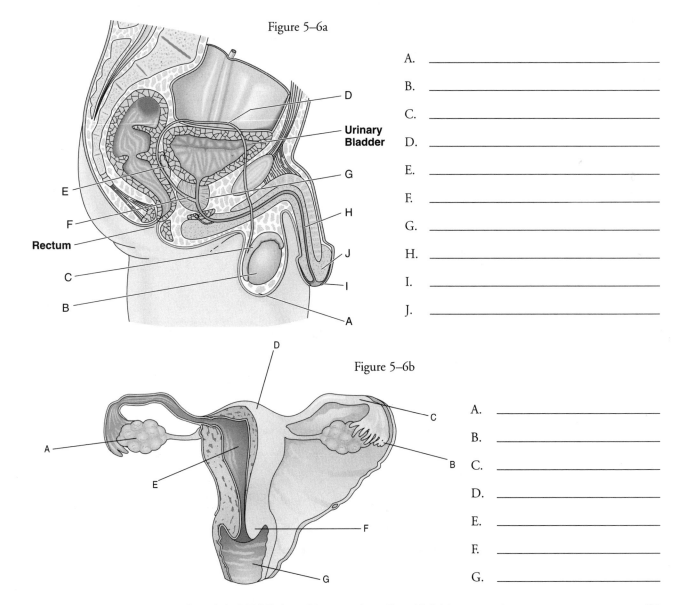

Figure 5–6a

A. _____
B. _____
C. _____
D. _____
E. _____
F. _____
G. _____
H. _____
I. _____
J. _____

Figure 5–6b

A. _____
B. _____
C. _____
D. _____
E. _____
F. _____
G. _____

CHAPTER 6 INFECTION CONTROL

Whenever an EMT-B approaches a sick or injured patient, there is a danger of contracting an infectious disease. For this reason, EMT-Bs must learn disease prevention and infection control.

Word Scramble: Unscramble the following words from the Key Terms found in Chapter 6 of the textbook.

1. tiumnonmziia _____

2. rrracie _____

3. aprxhpylios _____

4. sinomisntsor _____

5. gtacnosuio _____

6. oopcmmsciromunum _____

7. biantody _____

8. ocrimmsinorga _____

9. trocve _____

10. zihaabrdo _____

Listing: A. List five examples of common illnesses and give their mode of transmission.

1.

2.

3.

4.

5.

B. Give two examples of standards designed to protect EMTs from disease.

1.

2.

True or False: Read each statement and decide if it is TRUE or FALSE. Place T or F on the line before each statement.

1. _____ EMTs are at risk from infectious diseases only when the patient is bleeding.

2. _____ EMTs can expose patients to infectious diseases.

3. _____ An infection is caused by microscopic living creatures.

4. _____ Transmission of disease between people occurs only by direct contact.

5. _____ In order for disease to occur, the strength of the disease must overcome the host's defenses.

6. _____ All infectious diseases have immunizations.

7. _____ The EMT must take Standard Precautions when caring for a patient.

8. _____ There are no barrier devices available for the eyes.

9. _____ All waste generated on a patient care scene is considered a biohazard.

10. _____ EMTs can become carriers of disease while not becoming sick themselves.

Definitions: Write the definitions of the following terms.

safety officer _____

biohazard _____

personal protective equipment _____

immunocompromised _____

infection control manual _____

risk profile _____

Identification: Check the appropriate behaviors in preventing infection.

_____ Ongoing health assessment of the EMT.

_____ Putting on gloves, gown, and mask before any patient encounter, and then removing what is unnecessary.

_____ Carrying spare gloves for use with multiple patients.

_____ Washing hands only if gloves are unavailable or ripped.

_____ Using goggles or safety glasses to protect the eyes.

_____ Putting on a mask only if you are close to a patient.

_____ Using a gown for imminent childbirth.

_____ Using latex gloves for handling body fluids, and vinyl gloves for patient contact.

Fill in the Blank: Complete the following sentences that describe putting on and removing personal protective equipment.

The EMT should first put on _____ and _____ protection. He should then put on the _____ if it is necessary. Assistance may be needed in _____ the _____ in back. Put the _____ on last. To remove the PPE, the EMT should go in _____ order. Remove the _____. Then reach back and _____ or _____ the ties of the _____. Turn it inside out and roll it into a ball. Last remove the _____ and _____ protection. Finally, _____ your hands.

Matching: Match the terms with their definitions:

1. ____ Blood-borne Pathogens Rule

2. ____ Centers for Disease Control

3. ____ high-level disinfection

4. ____ intermediate-level disinfection

5. ____ infection control manual

6. ____ OSHA

7. ____ National Fire Protection Association

8. ____ sterilization

9. ____ Ryan White Law

10. ____ risk management

a. set of rules for employers regarding infection control practices

b. wiping down the surface with an EPA germicide or bleach solution

c. document that lists infection prevention procedures

d. requirement of hospitals to notify an EMS agency of a potential exposure to infectious disease

e. actions geared toward protection from infectious disease

f. federal organization that monitors transmission of infection

g. federal organization that sets association standards for preventing on-the-job illness or injury

h. required for equipment that touches a patient's mucous membranes

i. organization which sets requirements for firefighters

j. thorough cleaning so that all microorganisms are removed

Identification: Place a check mark in front of each of the following diseases that have an immunization available.

_____ AIDS   _____ rubella

_____ tuberculosis   _____ tetanus

_____ hepatitis B   _____ measles

Identification: State whether each of the following is an airborne, contact, vehicle, or vector-borne transmission by writing the correct word on the line in front.

1. _____ An EMT with a cold sneezes near another person who inhales the droplets.

2. _____ A paramedic eats food contaminated with salmonella.

3. _____ A paramedic accidentally sticks himself with a bloody needle.

4. _____ An EMT drinks contaminated water and develops diarrhea.

5. _____ A tick bites a child who becomes sick.

6. _____ A nurse develops a tear in her glove and blood enters an open cut.

7. _____ The paramedic touches dried blood on a stretcher and becomes ill.

8. _____ A patient coughs near the EMT who has not yet donned a mask.

Short Answer: Explain how hand washing is the single most important act in preventing the spread of infectious diseases.

Critical Thinking: Read the following case study and answer the questions after it.

Jess and Stephanie responded to a "man injured" while he was cutting shrubbery. Upon their arrival, they put on their gloves and proceeded to assess their patient, Mr. Ricci. He was alert but scared, and bleeding profusely from arm and hand injuries caused by electric shrub shears. Stephanie proceeded to care for the bleeding while Jess ensured that the shears were turned off and moved out of the way. While Stephanie and Jess assisted Mr. Ricci to the ambulance, Jess noticed that her glove had a jagged rip and the skin underneath was scraped.

1. What should Jess do now?

2. How can Jess accomplish this?

3. What should she do next?

4. Jess has been directed to see a physician while at the Emergency Department. Why is this necessary?

Student Name _____   Date _____

Skill 6–1: Hand Washing

Equipment Needed:

1. Liquid soap
2. Paper hand towels
3. Sink

Yes: ❑   Reteach: ❑   Return: ❑   Instructor initials: _____

Step One: Turn on the water and adjust it to a comfortable temperature. The water should flow freely.

Yes: ❑   Reteach: ❑   Return: ❑   Instructor initials: _____

Step Two: Liberally apply the liquid soap. Bar soap should be avoided because this type of soap harbors bacteria.

Yes: ❑   Reteach: ❑   Return: ❑   Instructor initials: _____

Step Three: Scrub vigorously, rubbing hands together to create friction. Particular attention should be paid to the space in between the fingers and the area under the nails. Skin underneath rings and watches should also be cleaned. Scrub for at least one minute.

Yes: ❑   Reteach: ❑   Return: ❑   Instructor initials: _____

Step Four: Rinse from wrists allowing soap and water to drip off fingertips.

Yes: ❑   Reteach: ❑   Return: ❑   Instructor initials: _____

Step Five: Dry hands with either a paper towel or air blower.

Yes: ❑   Reteach: ❑   Return: ❑   Instructor initials: _____

Step Six: Turn off faucet with clean towel.

Yes: ❑   Reteach: ❑   Return: ❑   Instructor initials: _____

Student Name _____ Date _____

Skill 6–2: Donning Gloves

Equipment Needed:

1. Nonsterile gloves
2. Hazardous waste container

Yes: ❑   Reteach: ❑   Return: ❑   Instructor initials: _____

Step One: Choose an appropriate size and type of glove for the task at hand.

Yes: ❑   Reteach: ❑   Return: ❑   Instructor initials: _____

Step Two: Arrange one glove so that the thumb is aligned with the thumb of the hand it is intended to go on.

Yes: ❑   Reteach: ❑   Return: ❑   Instructor initials: _____

Step Three: Grasp the front of the cuff with one hand, while sliding the other hand into the glove. Be sure to place each finger within the appropriate finger section.

Yes: ❑   Reteach: ❑   Return: ❑   Instructor initials: _____

Step Four: Pull at the cuff to ensure that the glove is completely applied to the hand.

Yes: ❑   Reteach: ❑   Return: ❑   Instructor initials: _____

Step Five: Repeat the process for the other hand.

Yes: ❑   Reteach: ❑   Return: ❑   Instructor initials: _____

Student Name _____   Date _____

Skill 6–3: Removal of Contaminated Gloves

Step One: Grasp the palm of the left glove with the gloved right hand.

Yes: ❑   Reteach: ❑   Return: ❑   Instructor initials: _____

Step Two: Pull the left glove toward the fingertips. The glove should turn inside out as it is removed.

Yes: ❑   Reteach: ❑   Return: ❑   Instructor initials: _____

Step Three: Hold the removed glove in the still gloved right hand.

Yes: ❑   Reteach: ❑   Return: ❑   Instructor initials: _____

Step Four: Place two fingers of the ungloved left hand under the cuff of the right glove, carefully avoiding any contaminated areas.

Yes: ❑   Reteach: ❑   Return: ❑   Instructor initials: _____

Step Five: Pull the right glove toward the fingertips, turning it inside out as it is removed.

Yes: ❑   Reteach: ❑   Return: ❑   Instructor initials: _____

Step Six: Completely remove the right glove, with the balled up left glove remaining inside the right glove as it is removed.

Yes: ❑   Reteach: ❑   Return: ❑   Instructor initials: _____

Step Seven: Dispose of the gloves in an approved biohazard container.

Yes: ❑   Reteach: ❑   Return: ❑   Instructor initials: _____

Step Eight: Wash hands thoroughly.

Yes: ❑   Reteach: ❑   Return: ❑   Instructor initials: _____

Student Name _____ Date _____

Skill 6–4: Donning a Gown and Mask

Equipment Needed:

1. Gown
2. Disposable mask
3. Hazardous waste container/laundry bin

Yes: ❏   Reteach: ❏   Return: ❏   Instructor initials: _____

Step One: Select an appropriate mask and eye protection for the task at hand.

Yes: ❏   Reteach: ❏   Return: ❏   Instructor initials: _____

Step Two: Fit the top of the mask to the bridge of the nose by squeezing on the flexible metal nosepiece within most masks.

Yes: ❏   Reteach: ❏   Return: ❏   Instructor initials: _____

Step Three: Pull the remainder of the mask to cover the chin. Ensure that the mask covers the nose and mouth with no gaps anywhere around the face, and that the eyes are not covered except by the transparent eye shield.

Yes: ❏   Reteach: ❏   Return: ❏   Instructor initials: _____

Step Four: Tie the mask ties at the top of the head and at the base of the skull to ensure a snug fit of the mask.

Yes: ❏   Reteach: ❏   Return: ❏   Instructor initials: _____

Step Five: If not a part of the chosen mask, apply appropriate eye protection.

Yes: ❏   Reteach: ❏   Return: ❏   Instructor initials: _____

Step Six: Select an appropriate gown for the task at hand.

Yes: ❏   Reteach: ❏   Return: ❏   Instructor initials: _____

Step Seven: Hold the gown up with the inside facing you and the top of the gown up.

Yes: ❏   Reteach: ❏   Return: ❏   Instructor initials: _____

(continues)

Skill 6–4: Continued

Step Eight: Place one arm then the other into the gown, pulling the neck of the gown up against your neck.

Yes: ❏   Reteach: ❏   Return: ❏   Instructor initials: _____

Step Nine: Reach around behind your neck and tie the neck ties snugly.

Yes: ❏   Reteach: ❏   Return: ❏   Instructor initials: _____

Step Ten: Reach around behind your waist and tie the waist ties snugly. If this is not feasible, ask a partner to tie the waist ties for you.

Yes: ❏   Reteach: ❏   Return: ❏   Instructor initials: _____

Student Name _____ Date _____

Skill 6–5: Removal of Contaminated Mask and Gown

Step One: After removal of contaminated gloves, the EMT should untie (or break if a paper gown) the waist and neck ties of the gown. If the gown is grossly contaminated, the EMT should ask a partner to do this to avoid contamination of his ungloved hands.

Yes: ❑   Reteach: ❑   Return: ❑   Instructor initials: _____

Step Two: With the left hand, grasp the right neckline of the gown, as close to the shoulder as possible without contamination, and pull the gown off the front of the body.

Yes: ❑   Reteach: ❑   Return: ❑   Instructor initials: _____

Step Three: As the gown is pulled forward, it should be removed from the right arm.

Yes: ❑   Reteach: ❑   Return: ❑   Instructor initials: _____

Step Four: The ungloved right hand can then grasp the uncontaminated inner surface of the gown and pull it off the left arm.

Yes: ❑   Reteach: ❑   Return: ❑   Instructor initials: _____

Step Five: Careful to touch only the uncontaminated inner surface of the gown, the EMT should roll the gown up and dispose of it in the appropriate hazardous waste container.

Yes: ❑   Reteach: ❑   Return: ❑   Instructor initials: _____

Step Six: Reaching behind the head, the EMT should untie, or tear, the ties from the mask.

Yes: ❑   Reteach: ❑   Return: ❑   Instructor initials: _____

Step Seven: The mask should be held by the uncontaminated ties and pulled away from the face.

Yes: ❑   Reteach: ❑   Return: ❑   Instructor initials: _____

Step Eight: The contaminated mask should be disposed of in the proper hazardous waste container.

Yes: ❑   Reteach: ❑   Return: ❑   Instructor initials: _____

CHAPTER 7 BASIC AIRWAY CONTROL

The human body needs oxygen in order for cells to produce energy. Oxygen gets into the body by first moving through the airway. Whenever a patient cannot keep his airway open, the EMT must keep it open.

Matching: Match word or words with the correct information. Place the letter of the correct information on the line in front of the term.

1. _____ esophagus
2. _____ mandible
3. _____ maxilla
4. _____ larynx
5. _____ nostrils
6. _____ pharynx
7. _____ uvula
8. _____ tonsils
9. _____ tongue
10. _____ epiglottis

a. upper jawbone
b. swings up to protect the nasal cavity
c. most common cause of airway obstruction
d. protects the top of the lower airway
e. pillars of fragile soft tissues in the throat
f. food passageway
g. voice box
h. lower jawbone
i. back of throat where oral and nasal cavities meet
j. openings to the nose from outside

Definition: Write the definition of each of the following terms.

ventilation _____

apnea _____

cyanosis _____

epiglottis _____

nasal flaring _____

sputum _____

sublingual _____

gag reflex _____

occlusion _____

Yankauer tip _____

Identification: Place a check mark in front of each word or phrase that is a sign or symptom of an obstructed or collapsed airway.

_____ apnea   _____ cough   _____ conjunctiva

_____ cyanosis   _____ snoring   _____ uvula

_____ breathlessness _____ intact dentures _____ sneezing

Ordering: Place the following steps to opening an airway of a noninjured patient in the correct order. Put a numeral 1 before the first step, 2 before the next, and so on.

_____ Maintain open airway during entire call

_____ Avoid pressure on underside of the jaw

_____ Kneel at the level of the head

_____ Push down on the forehead and lift up on the chin

_____ Place the palm of one hand on the forehead, and the fingertips on the jaw

Identification: Each of the following patients is in need of an airway assistive device; either an oropharyngeal airway (OPA), or a nasopharyngeal airway (NPA). Read each and then place the name of the correct device on the line in front of each scenario.

_____ The patient gagged when he was orally suctioned

_____ An unconscious patient

_____ A patient having a seizure who has clenched his teeth

_____ The patient was bleeding profusely from his nose

_____ There was no gag reflex with a fingersweep

_____ The patient's wife states that he has a history of nasal bleeding

_____ The patient has a large amount of soft palate damage

Correcting: Each of the following sentences is FALSE. Rewrite it as a correct statement.

1. Suctioning removes just fluids.

2. Suction, secure, open, and assess the airway.

3. Suction as deeply as the catheter will go.

4. Adequate suctioning will take 20-30 seconds.

5. Apply suction while advancing the catheter.

6. Use a French catheter to suction blood.

7. Yankauer catheters are best used for suctioning a tracheostomy.

8. Measure the depth of suctioning from the tip of the nose to the corner of the mouth.

9. Change suction catheters between each suction attempt.

10. It is not necessary to wear gloves when suctioning.

Critical Thinking: Read the following case study and then answer the questions.

Tania and Geoff are called to Castings Manufacturing Co. for a worker found unconscious next to his machine. The worker, John Wojtiak, is a 56-year-old man who has worked at the plant for 20 years. None of his coworkers heard or saw what happened.

1. What essential pieces of equipment must the EMTs bring to John's side?

2. What must Tania and Geoff do before using that equipment?

Upon arriving at Mr. Wojtiak's side, the EMTs find him lying on his back, snoring. They put on their PPE and begin to care for him.

3. What two signs point to a need to open the airway?

4. What method should Geoff choose to open the airway? Why?

5. What should be done next for the airway?

6. What airway assistive device should Tania place?

Following initial assessment and care, Mr. Wojtiak is placed on a backboard and a stretcher for transport to the hospital. Geoff provides care during the trip.

7. What important function must Geoff monitor and care for during the trip to the hospital? Why?

Student Name _____   Date _____

Skill 7–1: Head-Tilt, Chin-Lift Maneuver

Equipment Needed:

1. Gloves
2. Goggles
3. Mask

Yes: ❑   Reteach: ❑   Return: ❑   Instructor initials: _____

Step One: After donning the appropriate PPE, the EMT should position himself at the side of the patient's head.

Yes: ❑   Reteach: ❑   Return: ❑   Instructor initials: _____

Step Two: The palm of one hand should be placed on the patient's forehead, and the fingertips of the other hand on the patient's jaw.

Yes: ❑   Reteach: ❑   Return: ❑   Instructor initials: _____

Step Three: The patient's head is tilted back using a firm pressure on the forehead. Care should be taken not to push backward on the jaw, as this will only force the patient's mouth closed.

Yes: ❑   Reteach: ❑   Return: ❑   Instructor initials: _____

Step Four: The jaw is then gently lifted up to pull the tongue off the back of the throat.

Yes: ❑   Reteach: ❑   Return: ❑   Instructor initials: _____

Student Name _____   Date _____

Skill 7–2: Jaw Thrust Maneuver

Equipment Needed:

1. Gloves
2. Goggles
3. Mask

Yes: ❑   Reteach: ❑   Return: ❑   Instructor initials: _____

Step One: After donning the appropriate PPE, the EMT should position himself above the patient's head.

Yes: ❑   Reteach: ❑   Return: ❑   Instructor initials: _____

Step Two: The EMT should place his middle and index fingers on the angles of the patient's jaw and his thumbs on the cheekbones.

Yes: ❑   Reteach: ❑   Return: ❑   Instructor initials: _____

Step Three: The middle and index fingers lift the jaw and the tongue up off of the back of the throat while avoiding any movement of the neck.

Yes: ❑   Reteach: ❑   Return: ❑   Instructor initials: _____

Student Name _____   Date _____

Skill 7–3: Oral Suctioning

Equipment Needed:

1. Gloves
2. Goggles
3. Mask
4. Suction machine
5. Tubing
6. Catheter
7. Water

Yes: ❏   Reteach: ❏   Return: ❏   Instructor initials: _____

Step One: After donning the appropriate PPE, the EMT should assemble the suction equipment and test it by placing a finger over the distal end of the tubing, or kinking the tubing to generate suction. Most portable suction machines should generate between 200 and 300 mm Hg of suction.

Yes: ❏   Reteach: ❏   Return: ❏   Instructor initials: _____

Step Two: Select the appropriate catheter and attach it firmly to the distal end of the tubing.

Yes: ❏   Reteach: ❏   Return: ❏   Instructor initials: _____

Step Three: The distance from the corner of the mouth to the angle of the jaw should be measured as an estimate of the distance the catheter should be placed into the patient's mouth. The EMT should never suction beyond where he can see.

Yes: ❏   Reteach: ❏   Return: ❏   Instructor initials: _____

Step Four: The EMT should use the cross-finger technique to open the patient's mouth. Start by crossing the thumb under the index finger and placing the thumb against the lower teeth and the index finger against the upper teeth.

Yes: ❏   Reteach: ❏   Return: ❏   Instructor initials: _____

Step Five: Spread the thumb and index finger apart to open the patient's mouth.

Yes: ❏   Reteach: ❏   Return: ❏   Instructor initials: _____

Step Six: The suction catheter should be guided into the patient's mouth, taking care to follow the curvature of the tongue and only advancing as far as can be easily seen (or as far as measured in advance).

Yes: ❏   Reteach: ❏   Return: ❏   Instructor initials: _____

(continues)

Skill 7–3: Continued

Step Seven: A finger can then be placed over the whistle port on the catheter to generate suction. Suction should be applied while the catheter is being removed from the mouth, and should never be allowed to remain constant for more than 10–15 seconds.

Yes: ❑   Reteach: ❑   Return: ❑   Instructor initials: _____

Step Eight: The patient should then be reassessed, oxygen reapplied, and the procedure repeated as necessary.

Yes: ❑   Reteach: ❑   Return: ❑   Instructor initials: _____

Student Name _____ Date _____

Skill 7–4: Insertion of the Oropharyngeal Airway

Equipment Needed:

1. Gloves
2. Goggles
3. Mask
4. Assortment of OPA sizes

Yes: ❑   Reteach: ❑   Return: ❑   Instructor initials: _____

Step One: After donning the appropriate PPE, the EMT should measure the patient for an OPA. The appropriate size OPA reaches from the corner of the mouth to the bottom of the earlobe.

Yes: ❑   Reteach: ❑   Return: ❑   Instructor initials: _____

Step Two: Using the cross-finger technique, the EMT should open the patient's mouth.

Yes: ❑   Reteach: ❑   Return: ❑   Instructor initials: _____

Step Three: The proper size OPA should be initially guided into the patient's mouth with the curvature facing the tongue and the tip against the top of the mouth.

Yes: ❑   Reteach: ❑   Return: ❑   Instructor initials: _____

Step Four: At about the halfway point, the OPA is then turned in a 180 degree arc and passed the rest of the way into the mouth, following the curvature of the tongue.

Yes: ❑   Reteach: ❑   Return: ❑   Instructor initials: _____

Step Five: The OPA should rest with the flange against the patient's lips.

Yes: ❑   Reteach: ❑   Return: ❑   Instructor initials: _____

Student Name _____ Date _____

Skill 7–5: Insertion of the Nasopharyngeal Airway

Equipment Needed:

1. Gloves
2. Goggles
3. Mask
4. Assortment of NPA sizes
5. Water-soluble lubricant

Yes: ❑   Reteach: ❑   Return: ❑   Instructor initials: _____

Step One: After donning the appropriate PPE, the EMT should measure an NPA for size. The properly sized NPA will reach from the nostril to the tip of the earlobe.

Yes: ❑   Reteach: ❑   Return: ❑   Instructor initials: _____

Step Two: The NPA should be generously lubricated with a water-soluble lubricant to ease placement.

Yes: ❑   Reteach: ❑   Return: ❑   Instructor initials: _____

Step Three: The EMT should select the nostril that is the largest, usually the right.

Yes: ❑   Reteach: ❑   Return: ❑   Instructor initials: _____

Step Four: The lubricated NPA should be placed into the nostril with the bevel facing the nasal septum (middle of the nose) to minimize trauma to this vascular area.

Yes: ❑   Reteach: ❑   Return: ❑   Instructor initials: _____

Step Five: The NPA should be smoothly advanced straight back into the nose until the flange rests against the nostril. Note that the direction of advancement is posterior toward the pharynx, not up into the vascular structures of the nose.

Yes: ❑   Reteach: ❑   Return: ❑   Instructor initials: _____

CHAPTER 8 RESPIRATORY SUPPORT

The public has come to expect that EMTs are the experts in the techniques of respiratory support.

Matching: Match each word with its definition. Place the letter of the correct definition on the line in front of the term.

1. _____ hypoxia
2. _____ contraindication
3. _____ air hunger
4. _____ apnea
5. _____ dentures
6. _____ hypoventilation
7. _____ dyspnea
8. _____ tripod position
9. _____ stoma
10. _____ emphysema
11. _____ indication
12. _____ regulator
13. _____ tachypnea
14. _____ palpate
15. _____ pulse oximeter

a. posture of those in respiratory distress
b. the feeling of difficulty breathing
c. a lung disease
d. reasons to do something
e. allows for oxygen flow in liters per minute
f. false teeth
g. insufficient body stores of oxygen
h. device that measures oxygen on red cells
i. to feel with one's hands
j. breathing faster than normal
k. bypassing warming and filtering to get air in
l. breathing slower or ineffectively
m. reasons not to do something
n. lack of breathing
o. hole created after laryngectomy

Identification: Read the definitions. Write the correct word or terms on the line.

1. _____ muscles in the neck and chest that aid in breathing
2. _____ to listen
3. _____ compresses the esophagus
4. _____ muscles between the ribs
5. _____ instillation of moisture
6. _____ area that does not participate in gas exchange
7. _____ a device placed in nose, delivers 25–44% oxygen
8. _____ device that delivers nearly 100% oxygen
9. _____ exhaling past partially closed lips when in distress
10. _____ surgical hole to enable effective ventilation

Identification: Place a check mark in front of each word or phrase that is a sign or symptom of respiratory distress.

____ seesaw breathing   ____ cricoid pressure   ____ tripod

____ air hunger   ____ apex   ____ uvula

____ pursed lip breathing   ____ accessory muscle use   ____ sneezing

Short Answer: Answer the following questions from your reading.

1. How much oxygen is normally contained in air?

2. What is ventilation?

3. What is oxygenation?

4. Can ventilation occur without oxygenation? Describe.

Naming: For each description, write the name of the device.

1. _____ clear, plastic dome shaped device, with an air cushion to provide a seal; may have a filter and an oxygen inlet port

2. _____ originated from an anesthesia bag; is self-inflating

3. _____ a device that runs on oxygen; has a trigger to operate and can be used by one person

4. _____ a clear mask with an oxygen reservoir; delivers high concentration oxygen when set at 10 lpm or greater

5. _____ a small "mask" that fits over a stoma

6. _____ blue and corrugated, designed for use on transports of greater than an hour

7. _____ oxygen is delivered via prongs to the nose

Short Answer: Explain the possible consequences of failing to follow each of these safety tips regarding the use of oxygen.

1. Smoking near oxygen tanks.

2. Allowing petroleum products near tanks or fittings.

3. Storing oxygen in extreme temperatures.

4. Using a modified regulator from another gas cylinder.

5. Leaving an oxygen tank unattended.

6. Placing a portable oxygen tank standing up.

Critical Thinking: Read the following case study and then answer the questions.

Chris and Danny had just arrived back at the station when they were called to a home several blocks away. The caller had stated that her father was "having a little difficulty breathing." When they entered the man's room, Danny hung back for a second and watched the man. Chris began interviewing the daughter.

1. What is Danny looking for?

2. What information will Chris miss by interviewing the daughter?

The father, Mr. Allen, was sitting bolt upright with his hands on his knees. When he tried to speak to his daughter, he could manage only one word per breath. Danny noted that when Mr. Allen exhaled, he blew air out as if he was blowing out a candle.

3. What are the terms used to describe the observations made by Danny?

4. What assessments should Danny and Chris make next?

Chris used his stethoscope to listen to Mr. Allen's lungs. He heard air moving in and out on both sides, but it was accompanied by high-pitched wheezing. He placed a pulse oximeter on Mr. Allen's finger while Danny set up an oxygen mask.

5. What is the term for listening with a stethoscope?

6. What do the EMTs know about Mr. Allen's breathing and lung status based on their exam so far?

Danny placed a nonrebreather mask with 10 lpm oxygen on Mr. Allen and called dispatch to request a paramedic to the scene.

7. What percentage of oxygen is delivered by a nonrebreather mask at 10 lpm?

8. What should be done next for the airway?

9. What airway assistive device should Danny place on Mr. Allen?

Student Name _____   Date _____

Skill 8–1: Oxygen Tank Assembly

Equipment Needed:

1. Oxygen tank
2. Regulator with washer
3. Oxygen wrench or key

Yes: ❏   Reteach: ❏   Return: ❏   Instructor initials: _____

Step One: After ensuring that there is no risk of fire hazard in the area, the EMT should confirm that the tank at hand contains oxygen. These tanks are green in color and have pins that only match to the oxygen regulator for safety.

Yes: ❏   Reteach: ❏   Return: ❏   Instructor initials: _____

Step Two: Using an oxygen wrench, the EMT should quickly open and close the oxygen tank by turning the device at the top of the tank counterclockwise, then again clockwise. This procedure, called "cracking the tank," blows out any dirt and dust in the outlet.

Yes: ❏   Reteach: ❏   Return: ❏   Instructor initials: _____

Step Three: The EMT should then mate the regulator to the oxygen tank, being sure to tightly seat the regulator. Often a plastic washer is needed for an airtight fit.

Yes: ❏   Reteach: ❏   Return: ❏   Instructor initials: _____

Step Four: The oxygen tank may now be safely opened by again turning the device at the top of the tank counterclockwise as far as it allows, then back one-quarter turn. The pressure within the tank should be noted at this time.

Yes: ❏   Reteach: ❏   Return: ❏   Instructor initials: _____

Step Five: The tank is now ready to be used in oxygen delivery. To adjust the liter flow rate, the EMT can turn the flow adjusting knob on the regulator in a counterclockwise motion until the desired liter flow appears.

Yes: ❏   Reteach: ❏   Return: ❏   Instructor initials: _____

Student Name _____ Date _____

Skill 8–2: Application of Nonrebreather Oxygen Mask

Purpose: To provide the patient with high flow oxygen.

Standard Precautions:
- Hand washing
- Gloves

Equipment Needed:

1. Oxygen tank
2. Regulator
3. Nonrebreather oxygen mask   Yes: ❑   Reteach: ❑   Return: ❑   Instructor initials: _____

Step One: First, the EMT must ensure that the oxygen tank and oxygen regulator are correctly assembled. The oxygen tank should have sufficient pressure to provide continuous oxygen flow.

Yes: ❑   Reteach: ❑   Return: ❑   Instructor initials: _____

Step Two: Then the EMT should choose the correct oxygen administration device. A nonrebreather oxygen mask is used when high concentrations of oxygen are desired.

Yes: ❑   Reteach: ❑   Return: ❑   Instructor initials: _____

Step Three: To use the nonrebreather oxygen mask, the EMT must attach the oxygen tubing to the regulator and turn on the regulator. The regulator should never be turned below 6 lpm.

Yes: ❑   Reteach: ❑   Return: ❑   Instructor initials: _____

Step Four: The EMT would then place his thumbs over the valve between the bag and the mask, permitting the bag to fill completely.

Yes: ❑   Reteach: ❑   Return: ❑   Instructor initials: _____

Step Five: Grasping the mask in one hand and the elastic band in the other, the EMT would seat the mask firmly on the bridge of the nose, and drape the elastic band around the head. The EMT should pinch the metal strap around the nose.

Yes: ❑   Reteach: ❑   Return: ❑   Instructor initials: _____

Step Six: The EMT would then adjust the liter flow to ensure that the oxygen bag is always at least one-half full.

Yes: ❑   Reteach: ❑   Return: ❑   Instructor initials: _____

Student Name _____ Date _____

Skill 8–3: Application of Nasal Cannula

Purpose: To provide the patient with oxygen.

Standard Precautions:
- Hand washing
- Gloves

Equipment Needed:

1. Oxygen tank
2. Regulator
3. Nasal cannula   Yes: ❑ Reteach: ❑ Return: ❑ Instructor initials: _____

Step One: First, the EMT must ensure that the oxygen tank and oxygen regulator are correctly assembled. The oxygen tank should have sufficient pressure to provide continuous oxygen flow.

Yes: ❑ Reteach: ❑ Return: ❑ Instructor initials: _____

Step Two: Then the EMT should choose the correct oxygen administration device. A nasal cannula is used when the patient can tolerate the nonrebreather oxygen mask, or when low concentrations of oxygen are desired.

Yes: ❑ Reteach: ❑ Return: ❑ Instructor initials: _____

Step Three: To use the nasal cannula, the EMT must attach the oxygen tubing to the regulator and turn on the regulator. As a rule, 4 to 6 lpm is sufficient. The regulator should never be turned above 6 lpm.

Yes: ❑ Reteach: ❑ Return: ❑ Instructor initials: _____

Step Four: The nasal prongs should be gently introduced into the nostrils, so that they appear to be lying on the floor of the nostril.

Yes: ❑ Reteach: ❑ Return: ❑ Instructor initials: _____

Step Five: The tubing should be draped over the ears and the tubing cinched loosely under the chin with the ring. The nasal cannula should not be draped over like a necklace; the danger of strangulation is too great.

Yes: ❑ Reteach: ❑ Return: ❑ Instructor initials: _____

Step Six: The EMT would then adjust the liter flow to ensure that the patient is receiving an adequate liter flow.

Yes: ❑ Reteach: ❑ Return: ❑ Instructor initials: _____

Student Name _____ Date _____

Skill 8–4: Use of a Pocket Mask

Equipment Needed:

1. Pocket mask with oxygen outlet
2. One-way valve
3. Oxygen tubing
4. Oxygen tank
5. Oxygen regulator

Yes: ❑   Reteach: ❑   Return: ❑   Instructor initials: _____

Step One: After donning appropriate PPE and properly managing the nonbreathing patient's airway, the EMT should assemble the pocket mask by attaching the one-way valve to the pocket mask itself.

Yes: ❑   Reteach: ❑   Return: ❑   Instructor initials: _____

Step Two: The pocket mask should be applied over the patient's mouth and nose, with the narrower nosepiece placed over the bridge of the nose.

Yes: ❑   Reteach: ❑   Return: ❑   Instructor initials: _____

Step Three: Situated above the patient's head, the EMT should place his thumbs facing toward the patient's feet on either side of the mask, using the length of each to hold the mask to the patient's face. The fingers of each hand can then be placed under the angle of the jaw, which should be raised up to bring the face snugly against the mask, while the head is extended backward to maintain an open airway.

Yes: ❑   Reteach: ❑   Return: ❑   Instructor initials: _____

In the case of suspected spinal injury, the fingers of both hands will grasp under the angle of the jaw and lift up toward the mask, with care taken not to extend the neck at all. While this requires a tighter grip on the mask and jaw than the maneuver that is done without spinal injury, it is important the EMT take care not to worsen any potential spinal injury by extending the neck.

Yes: ❑   Reteach: ❑   Return: ❑   Instructor initials: _____

An airtight mask seal is crucial to effective ventilation via this method. The sound of air leaking means that air is not getting into the patient's lungs.

Yes: ❑   Reteach: ❑   Return: ❑   Instructor initials: _____

(continues)

Skill 8–4: Continued

Step Four: In order to ventilate the patient, the EMT should seal his lips around the ventilation port on the one-way valve and blow steadily into the port for 1½ to 2 seconds, or until the patient's chest is seen to rise. This should be repeated every 5 seconds for an adult, every 4 seconds for a child and every 3 seconds for an infant. Keep in mind that when ventilating smaller adults, children, and certainly infants, the volumes of air necessary to result in chest rise (and lung inflation) are much smaller. It is important to avoid causing overdistension of the lungs.

Yes: ❑   Reteach: ❑   Return: ❑   Instructor initials: _____

Step Five: Once the EMT has ventilated the patient for around 1 minute, it is important to recheck the status of pulse and respirations as in the quick check. At this time the EMT can also quickly turn on the oxygen tank, attach oxygen tubing to the pocket mask inlet, and run the oxygen at 15 lpm to deliver supplemental oxygen with each ventilation.

Yes: ❑   Reteach: ❑   Return: ❑   Instructor initials: _____

Step Six: With the supplemental oxygen attached, the EMT can return to ventilating the patient as previously described, rechecking the patient's status every few minutes.

Yes: ❑   Reteach: ❑   Return: ❑   Instructor initials: _____

Student Name _____ Date _____

Skill 8–5: Ventilation with a Bag-Valve-Mask Assembly

Equipment Needed:

1. Appropriate PPE (gloves, mask, goggles)
2. Bag-valve-mask (BVM) assembly
3. Oxygen tubing
4. Oxygen regulator
5. Oxygen tank

Yes: ❏   Reteach: ❏   Return: ❏   Instructor initials: _____

Step One: After applying appropriate PPE, the EMT must ensure that the oxygen tank and oxygen regulator are correctly assembled. The oxygen tank should have sufficient pressure to provide continuous oxygen flow.

Yes: ❏   Reteach: ❏   Return: ❏   Instructor initials: _____

Step Two: The EMT should then choose the correct oxygen administration device. A BVM assembly is used when an apneic patient needs to be ventilated by two EMTs.

Yes: ❏   Reteach: ❏   Return: ❏   Instructor initials: _____

Step Three: To use the BVM, the EMT must first attach the oxgen tubing to the regulator and turn on the regulator. As a rule, 10 to 15 lpm are sufficient.

Yes: ❏   Reteach: ❏   Return: ❏   Instructor initials: _____

Step Four: The EMT should choose a properly fitting facemask. The facemask should fit securely over the bridge of the nose and extend to the cleft of the chin.

Yes: ❏   Reteach: ❏   Return: ❏   Instructor initials: _____

Step Five: Ensuring that the airway has been opened, and an oral airway is in place, the EMT should place the mask over the apneic patient's face, maintaining the airway in an open position with either the jaw thrust or the head-tilt, chin-lift.

Yes: ❏   Reteach: ❏   Return: ❏   Instructor initials: _____

Step Six: One EMT should hold the mask in place, ensuring a good seal, while another EMT compresses the bag with two hands until chest rise is seen. The patient should be ventilated every 5 seconds.

Yes: ❏   Reteach: ❏   Return: ❏   Instructor initials: _____

Student Name _____   Date _____

Skill 8–6: Ventilation with a Flow-Restricted, Oxygen-Powered Ventilation Device

Equipment Needed:

1. Appropriate PPE
2. Flow-restricted, oxygen-powered ventilation device (FROPVD)
3. Oxygen regulator
4. Oxygen tank

Yes: ❏   Reteach: ❏   Return: ❏   Instructor initials: _____

Step One: The EMT must first ensure that the oxygen tank and oxygen regulator, with the FROPVD, are correctly assembled. The oxygen tank should show sufficient pressure to provide continuous oxygen flow.

Yes: ❏   Reteach: ❏   Return: ❏   Instructor initials: _____

Step Two: The EMT should then choose the correct oxygen administration device. An FROPVD is used when an apneic patient needs to be ventilated by an EMT.

Yes: ❏   Reteach: ❏   Return: ❏   Instructor initials: _____

Step Three: The EMT should then choose a properly fitting facemask. The facemask should fit securely over the bridge of the nose and extend to the cleft of the chin.

Yes: ❏   Reteach: ❏   Return: ❏   Instructor initials: _____

Step Four: Ensuring that the airway has been opened, and an oral airway is in place, the EMT should place the mask over the apneic patient's face, maintaining the airway in an open position with either the jaw thrust or the head-tilt, chin-lift.

Yes: ❏   Reteach: ❏   Return: ❏   Instructor initials: _____

Step Five: The EMT should then hold the mask in place while compressing the trigger of the FROPVD for about two seconds, or until the chest rises. The patient should be ventilated every 5 seconds.

Yes: ❏   Reteach: ❏   Return: ❏   Instructor initials: _____

CHAPTER 9 ADVANCED AIRWAY CONTROL

For a patient in need of extended airway maintenance, more secure means of stabilization may be required.

Identification: Place a check mark in front of each patient requiring endotracheal intubation by the trained EMT-B.

_____ An unconscious patient in respiratory distress with an OPA in place

_____ A patient who states that it hurts to breathe

_____ A pulseless and apneic patient

_____ An unresponsive patient who has taken an overdose of narcotics

_____ A seizing patient with a paramedic expected to arrive in 5 minutes

_____ A patient who is choking on meat but is coughing forcefully

_____ A patient with facial injuries who has gagged on an OPA

_____ Driver in a car versus tree collision; CPR in progress

Matching: Match the piece of equipment with its description.

1. ____ gloves, mask, eye protection
2. ____ orogastric tube
3. ____ end tidal CO_2 detector
4. ____ oxygen tank
5. ____ nasogastric tube
6. ____ laryngoscope handle
7. ____ Macintosh blade
8. ____ Miller blade
9. ____ ET tube
10. ____ stylet
11. ____ syringe
12. ____ OPA
13. ____ cuff
14. ____ Murphy eye

a. straight larygoscope blade
b. plastic tube placed in nose to stomach
c. opening on side of distal end of ET tube
d. rigid guide placed in ET tube
e. curved laryngoscope blade
f. plastic tube placed in mouth to stomach
g. plastic tube placed in the trachea
h. holds the batteries for direct laryngoscopy
i. inserts air into cuff
j. maintains seal when inflated
k. helps prevent infection
l. holds medicinal gas
m. indicates pressure of carbon dioxide
n. may be used as a bite block

Definitions: Write the correct definition of the term or phrase in the space following.

1. pneumothorax _____

2. hyperventilate _____

3. aspiration _____

4. tension pneumothorax _____

5. direct laryngoscopy _____

6. endotracheal intubation _____

True or False: Read each statement and decide if it is TRUE or FALSE. Place T or F on line before each statement.

1. _____ The vallecula is tissue covering the larynx.

2. _____ A cartilaginous flap of tissue at the base of the tongue is the epiglottis.

3. _____ The trachea connects the bronchii and the larynx.

4. _____ The upper jaw is the mandible.

5. _____ The opening at the vocal cords is the narrowest part of a child's airway.

6. _____ Cricoid pressure closes the epiglottis.

7. _____ The cricoid ring is the narrowest part of an adult's airway.

8. _____ Sniffing position is when the head is pushed forward toward the chest.

9. _____ The tongue must be moved to the right side of the mouth for endotracheal intubation.

10. _____ The carina is the point of bifurcation of the mainstem bronchii.

Ordering: Place the following actions in the order in which they should be performed for endotracheal intubation. Put a numeral 1 before the first action, a 2 before the next, and so on.

_____ Assess patient

_____ Lift blade upward and visualize the cords

_____ Ventilate and confirm placement

_____ Place distal end of tube through the opening between the cords

_____ Secure tube and reassess patient

_____ Assemble and test equipment

_____ Place OPA and hyperventilate the patient

_____ Remove blade

_____ Place blade into right side of patient's mouth and sweep the tongue left

_____ Lubricate and place stylet

_____ Place patient in sniffing position (provided there is no trauma)

_____ Stop ventilation

_____ Instill air into the pilot balloon and remove syringe

Short Answer: Describe how each method of tube placement confirmation works.

1. Visualization

2. Auscultation

3. Aspirator

4. CO$_2$ detector

5. Patient assessment

Short Answer: Describe how to correct each of the following situations during or after intubation.

1. What do the letters "DOPE" stand for in relation to ETT?

2. Upon auscultation, air movement is detected over the stomach. There is no chest rise.

3. The pilot balloon will not hold air and the patient can make sounds around the tube.

4. The stylet protrudes beyond the Murphy eye.

5. There are good breath sounds over the right lung but none over the left lung.

Critical Thinking 1: Read the following case study and answer the questions after it.

Luke, Maria, and Chris were called to the home of Mr. King, a middle-aged man with a history of respiratory difficulties. While assessing the patient and setting up equipment, Mr. King stopped breathing.

1. What should the EMTs do?

While Maria and Chris were completing the BLS tasks, Luke contacted their dispatcher. A paramedic unit was dispatched to the scene and would arrive in 3–5 minutes.

2. What should Maria and Chris do now?

3. What information should be given to the paramedics upon their arrival?

4. What equipment should be ready for the paramedics?

Critical Thinking 2: Read the following case study and answer the questions after it.

Denise and Steve were just completing a standby at the ski center located 45 minutes from the nearest hospital, when they were sent to a skier versus tree. The young man had struck the tree at a high rate of speed, and was lying supine on the snowy slope. Bystanders had taken C-spine stabilization and were waiting for the EMTs. The young man was making snoring and gurgling noises.

1. What should Denise and Steve do now?

While continuing their assessment, the young man stopped breathing.

2. How should Denise and Steve manage the young man's airway?

3. Describe the process they should use to properly manage it.

Student Name _____ Date _____

Skill 9–1: Assembly of Laryngoscope and Blade

Equipment Needed:

1. Appropriate PPE
2. Laryngoscope handle
3. Variety of blade types and sizes
4. Spare lightbulbs and batteries

Yes: ❑   Reteach: ❑   Return: ❑   Instructor initials: _____

Step One: The proximal end of the blade has a notched end that fits onto the handle securely.

Yes: ❑   Reteach: ❑   Return: ❑   Instructor initials: _____

Step Two: The notched end of the blade should be firmly attached to the handle with the blade in a closed position.

Yes: ❑   Reteach: ❑   Return: ❑   Instructor initials: _____

Step Three: Once properly attached, the blade can be extended, and the light bulb at its distal end should turn on.

Yes: ❑   Reteach: ❑   Return: ❑   Instructor initials: _____

Step Four: The bulb should quickly be checked for security in position (be sure it is tightly screwed on), and bright quality of light. If the light is dim, the bulb may be poorly connected, or the batteries may be low. It is the EMT's responsibility at the beginning of a shift to check the handles and blades to be sure they are functioning optimally.

Yes: ❑   Reteach: ❑   Return: ❑   Instructor initials: _____

Student Name _____ Date _____

Skill 9–2: Endotracheal Intubation

Equipment Needed:

1. Gloves
2. Mask
3. Eye protection
4. Suction unit
5. Yankauer catheters
6. Oxygen source
7. Bag-valve-mask device
8. Laryngoscope handle
9. Laryngoscope blades
10. Endotracheal tubes (different sizes)
11. Stylet
12. 10 cc syringe
13. Oropharyngeal airway
14. Tape or other securing device

Yes: ❑   Reteach: ❑   Return: ❑   Instructor initials: _____

Step One: The EMT who will be intubating should be above the head of the patient with the lit laryngoscope in his left hand, and the prepared endotracheal tube and suction catheter within reach of his right hand.

Yes: ❑   Reteach: ❑   Return: ❑   Instructor initials: _____

Step Two: Ventilation must be discontinued. The intubating EMT then places the patient's head in a sniffing position (assuming no spinal injury) and uses his right hand to open the patient's mouth, removing the OPA and any remaining dentures. An assisting provider should be applying gentle cricoid pressure.

Yes: ❑   Reteach: ❑   Return: ❑   Instructor initials: _____

Step Three: The larynogoscope blade should be placed into the right side of the patient's mouth and slid gently into the pharynx.

Yes: ❑   Reteach: ❑   Return: ❑   Instructor initials: _____

Step Four: The blade should be swept toward the patient's left, moving the tongue out of the visual field.

Yes: ❑   Reteach: ❑   Return: ❑   Instructor initials: _____

Step Five: The EMT should then lift the laryngoscope upward in order to move the patient's mandible out of the view. (Care should be taken not to allow the left wrist to bend and cause pressure from the laryngoscope on the upper teeth. Unnecessary pressure on the upper teeth can result in broken teeth that can then become airway foreign bodies and might also lead to an untoward cosmetic result.)

Yes: ❑   Reteach: ❑   Return: ❑   Instructor initials: _____

(continues)

Skill 9–2: Continued

Step Six: This maneuver should lift the upper airway structures out of the way and the EMT should be able to visualize the vocal cords and trachea. It should be noted that the trachea is the most anterior hollow structure and the esophagus is the most posterior. Suction should be used to clear any obstructing liquids for better visualization.

Yes: ❑   Reteach: ❑   Return: ❑   Instructor initials: _____

Step Seven: Once the triangular shaped, white-pink vocal cords have been visualized, the EMT should pick up the preformed tube with his right hand and place the distal end through the cords. (It is very important to continue to visualize the tube as it passes through the cords and into the trachea to avoid inadvertent misplacement.)

Yes: ❑   Reteach: ❑   Return: ❑   Instructor initials: _____

Step Eight: The tube should be advanced until the distal cuff is just past the vocal cords. (Or until the heavy black line at the distal end of an uncuffed pediatric tube has passed the cords.)

Yes: ❑   Reteach: ❑   Return: ❑   Instructor initials: _____

Step Nine: The EMT should then hold the tube in that position with his right hand while removing the laryngoscope from the patient's mouth with his left.

Yes: ❑   Reteach: ❑   Return: ❑   Instructor initials: _____

Step Ten: The left hand should then grasp the stylet and remove it from the endotracheal tube, careful not to displace the tube in the process.

Yes: ❑   Reteach: ❑   Return: ❑   Instructor initials: _____

Step Eleven: While maintaining a constant grip on the tube itself, the EMT should then pick up the syringe (which should still be attached to the pilot balloon at the proximal end of the tube) and instill 5–10 cc or air. (When the pilot balloon is full but still easily compressed, the right amount of air has been instilled and the distal cuff will be adequately inflated.)

Yes: ❑   Reteach: ❑   Return: ❑   Instructor initials: _____

Step Twelve: Once the cuff is inflated, the syringe should be removed from the pilot balloon to prevent inadvertent withdrawal of air. The syringe should be kept at hand, however, in case there is a need to readjust the tube position.

Yes: ❑   Reteach: ❑   Return: ❑   Instructor initials: _____

Step Thirteen: The placement of the tube should then be assessed, and once confimed to be in the trachea, it should be secured in place and the patient ventilated.

Yes: ❑   Reteach: ❑   Return: ❑   Instructor initials: _____

Chapter 10 A State of Hypoperfusion

Cells in the body require oxygen to function properly. When they are without oxygen for a period of time they will not be able to function and will eventually die. The EMT-B must be able to recognize compensated shock and set management priorities.

Fill In: Complete each line by choosing the correct word or phrase from the Key Terms found in Chapter 10 of the textbook.

```
         H _ _ _ _ _ _ _ _ _ _  _ _ _ _ _
           _ Y _ _ _ _ _ _ _ _
             P _ _ _
         _ _ _ O _ _ _ _ _ _ _ _
       _ _ _ _ _ P _ _ _ _ _ _ _
               E _ _ _ _ _ _ _ _ _ _ _
       _ _ _ _ _ _ R _ _ _ _ _  _ _ _ _
           _ _ _ F _ _ _ _ _
               U _ _ _ _ _ _ _ _ _
       _ _ _ _ _ _ S _ _ _ _
         _ _ _ _ I _ _ _ _ _ _ _  _ _ _ _
     _ _ _ _ _ _ _ O _ _ _ _ _ _
       _ _ _ _ _ _ _ N _ _  _ _ _ _ _
```

Fill in the Blank: Complete the circuit of blood throughout the body by filling in the correct word in each space.

Starting at the heart, the blood enters the _____, the largest artery in the body. It has many branches that serve head, chest, and abdomen. These branch further into smaller arteries called _____. These vessels contain _____ muscle which allows the vessels to change their diameter. Individual cells are served by the smallest of vessels called _____. These smallest vessels and the surrounding tissues are the _____ _____. Here, nutrients and oxygen are delivered to cells, and waste products are removed. Blood returns to the heart first by _____, then _____, and finally into the _____ _____, which returns deoxygenated blood to the heart. From there, the blood is sent to the lungs to be oxygenated and to begin another trip around the body.

Calculation: Calculate the cardiac output in each of the following cases, then answer the questions at the end. Use this formula: Cardiac output = stroke volume × heart rate

1. A patient has a stroke volume of 70 cc and a heart rate of 80 beats per minute.

2. A patient has a stroke volume of 70 cc and a heart rate of 40 beats per minute.

3. A patient has a stroke volume of 40 cc and a heart rate of 130 beats per minute.

4. Which patient has the best cardiac output?

5. What does this mean for individual cells?

6. Why do you think the stroke volume dropped when the heart rate went up?

Identification: Read the following and determine the type of shock in each case. Write the type on the line in front of the case.

1. _____ A patient bleeds profusely.

2. _____ A child has excessive nausea, vomiting, and diarrhea.

3. _____ A diabetic patient has an excessive amount of urination.

4. _____ A runner sweats profusely.

5. _____ A child, allergic to nuts, eats peanut brittle.

6. _____ A patient has a bacterial infection.

7. _____ A patient is stung by a wasp.

8. _____ A patient falls from a ladder onto his back.

9. _____ A patient develops a severe heart attack.

Ordering: Place in order from the first organ to lose perfusion to the last. Place a numeral 1 before the first, 2 before the next, and so on.

_____ brain _____ skin, muscles, bones, and uterus

_____ abdominal organs _____ heart and lungs

Identification: Read each set of signs/symptoms for an adult patient and decide if the set describes compensated or decompensated shock. Write the correct answer on the line in front of each.

1. _____ Pale, respiratory rate elevated, BP normal

2. _____ Cold, gray, unconscious, can't hear BP

3. _____ Confused, rapid pulse, BP low

4. _____ Anxious, BP normal, very fast pulse

5. _____ Thirsty, strong pulses at the wrist

6. _____ Nauseous, fast respirations, BP normal

7. _____ Agitated, BP normal, cool, pale

8. _____ No pulses at wrist, can't hear BP, cool

True or False: Read each statement and decide if it is TRUE or FALSE. Place T or F on line before each statement.

1. _____ Perfusion describes bringing oxygen into the lungs.

2. _____ Hypoperfusion means delivery of oxygenated blood to tissues is less than is necessary or not occurring.

3. _____ Lymph is the fluid part of the cardiovascular system.

4. _____ Capillaries can alter their diameter by contraction or relaxation of muscles.

5. _____ Increased respiratory rate is one of the body's compensatory mechanisms.

6. _____ Once the systolic BP drops to less than 90 mm Hg, irreversible shock results.

7. _____ As perfusion to the skin decreases, capillary refill time will increase.

8. _____ It is not necessary to reassess a patient's mental status, beyond that done initially.

9. _____ A drop in blood pressure associated with a change in position is called a positive tilt test.

10. _____ Use of the PSAG (MAST) is contraindicated in pelvic fractures.

Short Answer: Answer each of the following questions from your reading.

1. Which type(s) of shock are caused by the inability of the blood vessels to constrict?

2. Which type(s) of shock are due to fluid loss?

3. Which type(s) of shock are caused by the inability of the heart to pump?

4. Should PASG (MAST) be removed by the EMT-B? Why or why not?

5. How often should a patient experiencing hypoperfusion be monitored?

Critical Thinking 1: Read each scenario and then answer the questions that follow.

Cindy and Paul arrived at the Reams home for the 6-month-old daughter who has a "stomach bug" according to her mother. The child, Brittiany, had been vomiting and having diarrhea for two days. Her mother had been trying to get her to drink small amounts of liquids, but called EMS when she noticed that there were no wet diapers. Cindy performed an initial assessment while Paul gathered a history.

1. What important observations must Cindy make at this time?

2. Why is the child's response to her mother an important observation?

3. Explain the normal blood pressure result.

4. How should Cindy and Paul proceed?

Critical Thinking 2: Read each scenario and then answer the questions that follow.

Mrs. Evers called EMS because she had been very weak and dizzy. She was afraid that she would fall and injure herself. When Julie and Serge arrived, they found Mrs. Evers lying on her couch, pale, cool, and clammy. Julie obtained a history while Serge performed an initial assessment and began treatment. Mrs. Evers had a history of arthritis. Her doctor had started her on a new medicine that could cause bleeding in the stomach. Julie discovered that Mrs. Evers had been vomiting some material that looked like old blood and that her stools (bowel movements) had been very dark.

1. In addition to the usual baseline vital signs, what added assessment might Julie and Serge want to obtain?

2. How should Julie and Serge treat Mrs. Evers?

Critical Thinking 3: Read each scenario and then answer the questions that follow.

Brenda and Jerry responded to an incident where a man had fallen from a porch roof approximately 6 feet off the ground. When they arrived, the man was lying on his back on the ground. He was flushed and had a number of raised reddened areas on his trunk and arms. He also was breathing fast, and a high pitched whistle was noted with each breath. A pulse could not be found at the wrist.

1. What is the likely cause of the inability to find a pulse at the wrists?

2. What are the raised reddened areas called?

3. What treatments should Brenda and Jerry provide?

Student Name _____   Date _____

Skill 10–1: Orthostatic Vital Signs

Equipment Needed:

1. Gloves
2. Stethoscope
3. Blood pressure cuff
4. Watch with second hand
5. Assistant

Yes: ❑   Reteach: ❑   Return: ❑   Instructor initials: _____

Step One: Obtain a full set of vital signs from the supine patient.

Yes: ❑   Reteach: ❑   Return: ❑   Instructor initials: _____

Step Two: Assist the patient to standing, with an assistant behind the patient.

Yes: ❑   Reteach: ❑   Return: ❑   Instructor initials: _____

Step Three: Repeat vital signs.

Yes: ❑   Reteach: ❑   Return: ❑   Instructor initials: _____

Step Four: Compare vital signs lying and standing.

Yes: ❑   Reteach: ❑   Return: ❑   Instructor initials: _____

Step Five: Treat for shock as indicated.

Yes: ❑   Reteach: ❑   Return: ❑   Instructor initials: _____

Step Six: Record or report significant changes.

Yes: ❑   Reteach: ❑   Return: ❑   Instructor initials: _____

Student Name _____   Date _____

Skill 10–2: Application of MAST

Equipment Needed:

1. Gloves
2. MAST with foot pump attached
3. Stethoscope
4. Blood pressure cuff

Yes: ❑   Reteach: ❑   Return: ❑   Instructor initials: _____

Step One: Perform initial assessment and vital signs.

Yes: ❑   Reteach: ❑   Return: ❑   Instructor initials: _____

Step Two: Identify indications for MAST application: injured patient with severe hypotension (SBP<50), or hypotension (SBP<90) with associated pelvic instability with other signs of shock (>2 of the following: altered mental status, persistent tachycardia, cool and clammy skin, diaphoresis, thirst, or nausea.)

Yes: ❑   Reteach: ❑   Return: ❑   Instructor initials: _____

Step Three: Ensure lack of absolute contraindications: pulmonary edema, or penetrating chest injury.

Yes: ❑   Reteach: ❑   Return: ❑   Instructor initials: _____

Step Four: Assess for relative contraindications: pregnancy, impaled object, evisceration.

Yes: ❑   Reteach: ❑   Return: ❑   Instructor initials: _____

Step Five: Apply trousers to patient's lower body. (Be sure not to allow trousers to cover ribcage at all.)

Yes: ❑   Reteach: ❑   Return: ❑   Instructor initials: _____

Step Six: Secure Velcro fasteners.

Yes: ❑   Reteach: ❑   Return: ❑   Instructor initials: _____

Step Seven: Attach air pump hoses and set to open position.

Yes: ❑   Reteach: ❑   Return: ❑   Instructor initials: _____

(continues)

Skill 10–2: Continued

Step Eight: Use foot pump to inflate trousers until gauge reaches 106 mm Hg or pop-offs release.

Yes: ❑   Reteach: ❑   Return: ❑   Instructor initials: _____

Step Nine: Set air pump hoses to closed position.

Yes: ❑   Reteach: ❑   Return: ❑   Instructor initials: _____

Step Ten: Reassess patient's ABCs and vital signs.

Yes: ❑   Reteach: ❑   Return: ❑   Instructor initials: _____

CHAPTER 11   BASELINE VITAL SIGNS AND SAMPLE HISTORY

During the course of training, the EMT-B will learn many skills. Those which will be utilized most frequently are obtaining vital signs and gathering a basic patient history.

Definitions: Define the following terms.

1. anisocoria   _____

2. cyanosis   _____

3. constricted   _____

4. jaundice   _____

5. dilated   _____

6. pallor   _____

7. diastolic   _____

8. PERRL   _____

9. systolic   _____

10. syphgmomenometer _____

Matching: Match the word or words with its definition. Place the letter of the correct definition on the line in front of the term.

1. _____ inspiration

2. _____ exhalation

3. _____ pulse oximeter

4. _____ stridor

5. _____ gurgling

6. _____ snoring

7. _____ wheezing

8. _____ grunting

9. _____ accessory muscles

10. _____ nasal flaring

a. nostrils opening widely with each breath

b. harsh inspiratory sound

c. noise caused by blockage with the tongue

d. neck and chest muscles

e. breathing in

f. high-pitched inspiratory or expiratory sound

g. device to measure oxygen on the RBCs

h. breathing out

i. noise from liquid in the airway

j. noise from extreme effort to breathe

Calculation: Calculate the following respiratory rates.

1. 15 breaths in 30 seconds = _____ breaths per minute

2. 10 breaths in 30 seconds = _____ breaths per minute

3. 24 breaths in 60 seconds = _____ breaths per minute

4. 6 breaths in 30 seconds = _____ breaths per minute

Calculation: Calculate the following pulse rates.

1. 32 beats in 30 seconds = _____ beats per minute

2. 45 beats in 30 seconds = _____ beats per minute

3. 68 beats in 60 seconds = _____ beats per minute

4. 90 beats in 60 seconds = _____ beats per minute

5. 52 beats in 30 seconds = _____ beats per minute

True or False: Read each statement and decide if it is TRUE or FALSE. Place T or F on line before each statement.

_____ The systolic pressure measures the heart at rest.

_____ Diastolic pressure measures force in the arteries during cardiac relaxation.

_____ A cuff that covers one third of the upper arm is the correct size.

_____ To auscultate a blood pressure, the EMT-B will need a stethoscope.

_____ Palpating a blood pressure is more accurate than auscultation.

Sorting: Complete the following table of skin signs by placing the descriptor in the column described.

cool   pallor

jaundice   hot

sweaty   cyanosis

flushed   gray

pink   warm

dry

Color	**Temperature**	**Condition**

Identification: Read each of the following and determine if it describes a sign or a symptom. Place the correct word on the line in front of the term.

1. _____ Pulse of 92 beats per minute

2. _____ "I can't breathe"

3. _____ Leg pain

4. _____ Tenderness when touched

5. _____ Accessory muscle use

6. _____ Grunting respirations

7. _____ Nausea

8. _____ Vomiting

9. _____ Cyanosis

10. _____ 22 breaths per minute

11. _____ Dizzy

12. _____ Chest pain

13. _____ Dry skin

14. _____ Sweaty

15. _____ Headache

Sorting: Read the following patient story. Place the information into the correct SAMPLE category.

Mr. Jones called EMS because he was having difficulty breathing. He sat in the tripod position and used accessory muscles to breathe. Normally, his inhaler of Ventolin helped but today it didn't. He wanted his doctor to order more medications but at present only had the inhaler. He was taking vitamins and a daily aspirin to help him feel better. His doctor had told him that he had lung disease caused by many years of smoking. Also, eggs caused him to break out in hives. He used his inhaler one hour before calling EMS, and had eaten breakfast that morning. The hot and humid weather always seemed to bother him.

S

A

M

P

L

E

Student Name _____ Date _____

Skill 11–1: Measurement of Respiration

Equipment Needed:

1. PPE (minimally gloves)
2. Watch/clock with second hand

Yes: ❑   Reteach: ❑   Return: ❑   Instructor initials: _____

Step One: Apply any appropriate personal protective equipment.

Yes: ❑   Reteach: ❑   Return: ❑   Instructor initials: _____

Step Two: Observe patient's chest or abdomen for rise and fall with respiration, noting any irregular patterns, noises, or effort.

Yes: ❑   Reteach: ❑   Return: ❑   Instructor initials: _____

Step Three: Note whether the respiration is shallow or particularly labored.

Yes: ❑   Reteach: ❑   Return: ❑   Instructor initials: _____

Step Four: Count the number of complete breaths taken (one inspiration and one exhalation counts as *one* breath) over a 30 second period.

Yes: ❑   Reteach: ❑   Return: ❑   Instructor initials: _____

Step Five: Multiply this number by 2 to obtain breaths per minute.

Yes: ❑   Reteach: ❑   Return: ❑   Instructor initials: _____

Step Six: Record the respiratory rate and quality.

Yes: ❑   Reteach: ❑   Return: ❑   Instructor initials: _____

Student Name _____ Date _____

Skill 11–2: Measurement of Pulse

Equipment Needed:

1. PPE (minimally gloves)
2. Watch/clock with second hand

Yes: ❑   Reteach: ❑   Return: ❑   Instructor initials: _____

Step One: Apply appropriate personal protective equipment.

Yes: ❑   Reteach: ❑   Return: ❑   Instructor initials: _____

Step Two: Find radial pulse at thumb side of wrist, and note the quality and regularity of the pulse.

Yes: ❑   Reteach: ❑   Return: ❑   Instructor initials: _____

Step Three: Count the number of pulse beats felt over a 30 second period.

Yes: ❑   Reteach: ❑   Return: ❑   Instructor initials: _____

Step Four: Multiply this number by 2 to obtain beats per minute.

Yes: ❑   Reteach: ❑   Return: ❑   Instructor initials: _____

Step Five: Record the pulse rate, quality, and regularity.

Yes: ❑   Reteach: ❑   Return: ❑   Instructor initials: _____

Student Name _____ Date _____

Skill 11–3: Measurement of Blood Pressure by Auscultation

Equipment Needed:

1. PPE (minimally gloves)
2. Stethoscope
3. Properly sized blood pressure cuff

Yes: ❑   Reteach: ❑   Return: ❑   Instructor initials: _____

Step One: Apply appropriate personal protective equipment.

Yes: ❑   Reteach: ❑   Return: ❑   Instructor initials: _____

Step Two: Place the blood pressure cuff snugly around the patient's upper arm.

Yes: ❑   Reteach: ❑   Return: ❑   Instructor initials: _____

Step Three: Find the brachial pulse.

Yes: ❑   Reteach: ❑   Return: ❑   Instructor initials: _____

Step Four: Close the valve on the cuff.

Yes: ❑   Reteach: ❑   Return: ❑   Instructor initials: _____

Step Five: Inflate the cuff until the brachial pulse is no longer felt, then 20 points higher.

Yes: ❑   Reteach: ❑   Return: ❑   Instructor initials: _____

Step Six: Place the stethoscope on the brachial pulse and in your ears.

Yes: ❑   Reteach: ❑   Return: ❑   Instructor initials: _____

Step Seven: Slowly deflate the blood pressure cuff using the valve next to the bulb.

Yes: ❑   Reteach: ❑   Return: ❑   Instructor initials: _____

Step Eight: Note the systolic and the diastolic pressures.

Yes: ❑   Reteach: ❑   Return: ❑   Instructor initials: _____

(continues)

Skill 11–3: Continued

Step Nine: Allow complete deflation of cuff.

Yes: ❑   Reteach: ❑   Return: ❑   Instructor initials: _____

Step Ten: Record blood pressure.

Yes: ❑   Reteach: ❑   Return: ❑   Instructor initials: _____

Student Name _____ Date _____

Skill 11–4: Measurement of Blood Pressure by Palpation

Equipment Needed:

1. PPE (minimally gloves)
2. Properly sized blood pressure cuff

Yes: ❑   Reteach: ❑   Return: ❑   Instructor initials: _____

Step One: Apply appropriate personal protective equipment.

Yes: ❑   Reteach: ❑   Return: ❑   Instructor initials: _____

Step Two: Place the blood pressure cuff snugly around the patient's upper arm.

Yes: ❑   Reteach: ❑   Return: ❑   Instructor initials: _____

Step Three: Find the radial pulse.

Yes: ❑   Reteach: ❑   Return: ❑   Instructor initials: _____

Step Four: Close the valve on the cuff.

Yes: ❑   Reteach: ❑   Return: ❑   Instructor initials: _____

Step Five: Inflate the cuff until the radial pulse is no longer felt, then 20 points higher.

Yes: ❑   Reteach: ❑   Return: ❑   Instructor initials: _____

Step Six: Slowly deflate the blood pressure cuff using the valve next to the bulb.

Yes: ❑   Reteach: ❑   Return: ❑   Instructor initials: _____

Step Seven: Note the pressure on the valve at the time that you feel the return of the radial pulse.

Yes: ❑   Reteach: ❑   Return: ❑   Instructor initials: _____

(continues)

Skill 11–4: Continued

Step Eight: Allow complete deflation of cuff.

Yes: ❏   Reteach: ❏   Return: ❏   Instructor initials: _____

Step Nine: Record blood pressure.

Yes: ❏   Reteach: ❏   Return: ❏   Instructor initials: _____

Student Name _____   Date _____

Skill 11–5: Pulse Oximetry

Equipment Needed:

1. Appropriate personal protective equipment
2. Pulse oximeter with indicator light
3. Nail polish remover

Yes: ❏   Reteach: ❏   Return: ❏   Instructor initials: _____

Step One: Apply appropriate personal protective equipment.

Yes: ❏   Reteach: ❏   Return: ❏   Instructor initials: _____

Step Two: Assess the patient and apply oxygen as thought appropriate.

Yes: ❏   Reteach: ❏   Return: ❏   Instructor initials: _____

Step Three: Turn on the pulse oximeter.

Yes: ❏   Reteach: ❏   Return: ❏   Instructor initials: _____

Step Four: Place probe on patient's finger (if nail polish is present, must remove polish first).

Yes: ❏   Reteach: ❏   Return: ❏   Instructor initials: _____

Step Five: Note indicator light assuring adequate sampling.

Yes: ❏   Reteach: ❏   Return: ❏   Instructor initials: _____

Step Six: Note reading as "percent saturated" and document it.

Yes: ❏   Reteach: ❏   Return: ❏   Instructor initials: _____

Step Seven: Turn device off and store in safe location.

Yes: ❏   Reteach: ❏   Return: ❏   Instructor initials: _____

CHAPTER 12 LIFTING AND MOVING PATIENTS

Packaging, lifting, and carrying occurs on every EMS call. It is one of the fundamental aspects of EMS that has not changed over time.

Definition: The following are methods for lifting and moving patients. Choose the correct one from the list and place it on the line.

arm drag

blanket drag

caterpillar pass

clothing drag

cradle carry

diamond stretcher carry

direct carry

direct lift

emergency moves

end-to-end stretcher carry

extremity carry

firefighter's carry

firefighter's drag

pack strap carry

power lift

rescuer assist

seat carry

squat lift

1. _____ A carry in which the patient's arms are around the EMT's neck and the EMT crawls with the patient's body underneath

2. _____ A technique used by a single EMT to help a patient to walk

3. _____ A method of movement in which the EMT-B grasps the patient's wrists and pulls the arms back over the patient's head

4. _____ A carry in which the EMT-B grasps the patient's arms and hoists the patient onto his back with the feet dragging

5. _____ A method of carrying a stretcher in which there is an EMT-B on each end plus one on each side

6. _____ A carry in which two EMT-Bs lock arms and allow the patient to sit on their arms

7. _____ Two EMT-Bs, one on each end of the stretcher, carry it

8. _____ A means to replace tired EMT-Bs with rested ones without lowering the stretcher

9. _____ Also called a power lift

10. _____ Technique that involves lifting a patient up onto the EMT-B's shoulders to quickly move him from a dangerous environment

11. _____ A technique used to lift a heavy object from the ground

12. _____ Use of collar or handful of clothing to quickly remove a patient from a dangerous scene

13. _____ A technique that allows three EMT-Bs to lift a patient from the ground without using assistive devices

14. _____ Methods that allow an EMT-B to rapidly remove a patient in an emergency

15. _____ Lifting a person and carrying him a short distance to a stretcher

16. _____ Placing a patient on a blanket and dragging it over the ground

17. _____ Holding a patient in one's arms and carrying him for a rapid move

18. _____ Two EMT-Bs lift the patient under arms and knees

Matching: Match the description of each device with its name by placing the correct letter on the line in front.

1. _____ flexible stretcher
2. _____ cravat
3. _____ draw sheet
4. _____ stairchair
5. _____ transfer board
6. _____ basket stretcher
7. _____ Reeves stretcher
8. _____ scoop stretcher

a. protection over rough terrain
b. sturdy linen for transferring a patient
c. plastic stretcher that rolls up when unused
d. commercial flexible stretcher
e. can be separated for placement
f. also called a slide board
g. triangular cotton dressing
h. with wheels for moving a seated patient

Identification: Read each scenario and decide which require an emergency move. Place a check on the line before those that require an emergency move.

1. _____ Person stuck in a car; complaining of leg pain
2. _____ Person unconscious from smoke in a fireworks factory
3. _____ Person with a fractured leg is lying across a patient in respiratory arrest
4. _____ The driver of a car smashed his face and knocked out several teeth; airway patent
5. _____ Person is still inside a vehicle which has overturned into a creek
6. _____ A person is complaining of back and leg pain
7. _____ A person has bleeding from a head laceration
8. _____ A person is complaining of mild shortness of breath following a fender bender
9. _____ A person collapses outside a building where there is a gas leak
10. _____ A person is in respiratory arrest following a minor accident

Short Answer: Answer each of the following questions regarding back care.

1. What region of the spine is likely to suffer an injury from improper lifting or moving?

2. Why do exercises help prevent back injury?

3. The EMT-B needs to lift the extrication tools from the floor. The tools weigh 45 pounds. Describe the correct way to lift them.

4. A patient must be moved onto a hospital stretcher. Describe two ways in which an EMT-B can accomplish this safely.

5. Deanna is afraid she will injure her back, so she has chosen to wear a back support tightly whenever she is on duty. Explain how this choice could actually cause Deanna to have an injury.

Critical Thinking: Read each scenario. Decide how to move the patient from scene to ambulance.

George, Jason, and Steve were called to the Johnson residence for Mrs. Johnson, who had fallen. Mrs. Johnson was a fiercely independent woman who took pride in running her small Mom and Pop grocery store, even at age 78. Upon their arrival, they found Mrs. Johnson lying on her right side in a cramped narrow aisle. She stated that she was turning around quickly, felt a "snap" at her hip, and couldn't stay standing. She lowered herself to the floor but now couldn't move due to the pain in her right leg and hip.

Corinne, Rebekah, and Tim answered a cell phone call for a "man down" at the local high school. Once there, they found Mr. Joli, the janitor. He said that he had been readying cleaners to really clean the area before graduation and had tripped over a bucket, falling forward onto his arms. His arms hurt, and his right leg was deformed and very painful. Worse, the chemicals had spilled and were very slowly running toward one another.

Ted and Katie are called to the third-floor walk-up of Mrs. Hedderman. They find her seated upright in a chair, having trouble breathing.

Student Name _____ Date _____

Skill 12–1: Proper Lifting Techniques

Equipment Needed:

1. Appropriate PPE
2. Appropriate back support
3. Proper footwear
4. Adequate numbers of trained assistants

Yes: ❑   Reteach: ❑   Return: ❑   Instructor initials: _____

Step One: The EMT should try to position his feet about shoulder length apart, facing forward.

Yes: ❑   Reteach: ❑   Return: ❑   Instructor initials: _____

Step Two: The EMT would then lower his body by bending at knees, one knee down, keeping back straight.

Yes: ❑   Reteach: ❑   Return: ❑   Instructor initials: _____

Step Three: Grasping object with hands, palms upward (power grip), the EMT would lift evenly and smoothly.

Yes: ❑   Reteach: ❑   Return: ❑   Instructor initials: _____

Step Four: With arms locked out straight, the EMT stands fully upright.

Yes: ❑   Reteach: ❑   Return: ❑   Instructor initials: _____

Student Name _____ Date _____

Skill 12–2: Clothing Drag

Equipment Needed:

1. Appropriate PPE

Yes: ❑   Reteach: ❑   Return: ❑   Instructor initials: _____

Step One: The EMT would grasp the patient's clothing at the collar, while cradling the patient's head on his forearms.

Yes: ❑   Reteach: ❑   Return: ❑   Instructor initials: _____

Step Two: Crouching down, with back straight, the EMT would walk backwards.

Yes: ❑   Reteach: ❑   Return: ❑   Instructor initials: _____

Student Name _____ Date _____

Skill 12–3: Arm Drag

Equipment Needed:

1. Appropriate PPE

Yes: ❏ Reteach: ❏ Return: ❏ Instructor initials: _____

Step One: Kneeling down, the EMT slides his arms under the patient's arms, grasps the wrists across the chest.

Yes: ❏ Reteach: ❏ Return: ❏ Instructor initials: _____

Step Two: Standing up, the EMT walks backwards.

Yes: ❏ Reteach: ❏ Return: ❏ Instructor initials: _____

Student Name _____ Date _____

Skill 12–4: Blanket Drag

Equipment Needed:

1. Appropriate PPE
2. Blanket, tarp, drape, or similar covering

Yes: ❏   Reteach: ❏   Return: ❏   Instructor initials: _____

Step One: Place the blanket along the long axis of the body, leaving about one foot of material at the head.

Yes: ❏   Reteach: ❏   Return: ❏   Instructor initials: _____

Step Two: Log roll the patient onto the blanket, pulling the blanket from underneath the patient.

Yes: ❏   Reteach: ❏   Return: ❏   Instructor initials: _____

Step Three: Wrap the patient with the blanket, protecting the patient.

Yes: ❏   Reteach: ❏   Return: ❏   Instructor initials: _____

Step Four: Roll up the excess material at the head and grasp the roll.

Yes: ❏   Reteach: ❏   Return: ❏   Instructor initials: _____

Student Name _____ Date _____

Skill 12–5: Firefighter's Drag

Equipment Needed:

1. Appropriate PPE
2. Triangular bandage

Yes: ❑   Reteach: ❑   Return: ❑   Instructor initials: _____

Step One: Using the triangular bandage, folded into a cravat, the EMT would secure the patient's wrists together.

Yes: ❑   Reteach: ❑   Return: ❑   Instructor initials: _____

Step Two: While on all fours, the EMT would drape the tied hands over his shoulders and drag the patient underneath him.

Yes: ❑   Reteach: ❑   Return: ❑   Instructor initials: _____

Student Name _____ Date _____

Skill 12–6: Rescuer Assist

Equipment Needed:

1. Appropriate PPE

Yes: ❑ Reteach: ❑ Return: ❑ Instructor initials: _____

Step One: The EMT would crouch to the patient's level, and swing one arm over the EMT's shoulders.

Yes: ❑ Reteach: ❑ Return: ❑ Instructor initials: _____

Step Two: With one hand grasping the patient's beltline, and another grasping the patient's other wrist, the EMT stands and assists the patient with walking.

Yes: ❑ Reteach: ❑ Return: ❑ Instructor initials: _____

Student Name _____   Date _____

Skill 12–7: Pack Strap Carry

Equipment Needed:

1. Appropriate PPE

Yes: ❑   Reteach: ❑   Return: ❑   Instructor initials: _____

Step One: Kneeling in front of the seated patient, grasp the patient's wrists and pivot on the heels, draping the patient's arms over the sholders.

Yes: ❑   Reteach: ❑   Return: ❑   Instructor initials: _____

Step Two: Stand and hoist the patient onto the shoulders and off his feet.

Yes: ❑   Reteach: ❑   Return: ❑   Instructor initials: _____

Student Name _____ Date _____

Skill 12–8: The Cradle Carry

Equipment Needed:

1. Appropriate PPE

Yes: ❑ Reteach: ❑ Return: ❑ Instructor initials: _____

Step One: The EMT would first kneel next to the supine patient, placing one hand under the shoulders and the other hand under the knees.

Yes: ❑ Reteach: ❑ Return: ❑ Instructor initials: _____

Step Two: The EMT would then stand, keeping the patient's body close to his. (Tying the hands together with a cravat helps with some of the work of carrying).

Yes: ❑ Reteach: ❑ Return: ❑ Instructor initials: _____

Student Name _____   Date _____

Skill 12–9: The Firefighter's Carry

Equipment Needed:

1. Appropriate PPE

Yes: ❏   Reteach: ❏   Return: ❏   Instructor initials: _____

Step One: The EMT starts by standing toe-to-toe with the supine patient. Crouching down, he grabs the patient's wrists and proceeds to roll the patient to a seated position.

Yes: ❏   Reteach: ❏   Return: ❏   Instructor initials: _____

Step Two: Without stopping, the EMT then pulls the patient as nearly erect as possible.

Yes: ❏   Reteach: ❏   Return: ❏   Instructor initials: _____

Step Three: Quickly crouching again, the EMT places his shoulder into the patient's abdomen, while simultaneously standing.

Yes: ❏   Reteach: ❏   Return: ❏   Instructor initials: _____

Step Four: The EMT would then put one arm throught the patient's legs and grasp the patient's hand lying across his chest, effectively locking the patient over his shoulders. (Another EMT may help hoist the patient up onto the shoulders of the EMT. The second EMT waits until the patient is up and over the first EMT's shoulders then, grasping the patient's knee, helps hoist the patient.)

Yes: ❏   Reteach: ❏   Return: ❏   Instructor initials: _____

Student Name _____ Date _____

Skill 12–10: The Seat Carry

Equipment Needed:

1. Appropriate PPE

Yes: ❏   Reteach: ❏   Return: ❏   Instructor initials: _____

Step One: The two EMTs kneel on opposite knees, and clasp arms. Each EMT should grasp the other EMT at the elbow.

Yes: ❏   Reteach: ❏   Return: ❏   Instructor initials: _____

Step Two: With one pair of arms low and one pair high, the patient sits back into the seat that has been created. The EMTs then stand together, at the same time.

Yes: ❏   Reteach: ❏   Return: ❏   Instructor initials: _____

Student Name _____   Date _____

Skill 12–11: The Chair Carry

Equipment Needed:

1. Appropriate PPE
2. Hardback chair

Yes: ❏   Reteach: ❏   Return: ❏   Instructor initials: _____

Step One: The patient is assisted to sitting in the chair.

Yes: ❏   Reteach: ❏   Return: ❏   Instructor initials: _____

Step Two: One EMT kneels in front of the chair, facing forward, and between the patient's legs. He reaches back and grasps the legs of the chair.

Yes: ❏   Reteach: ❏   Return: ❏   Instructor initials: _____

Step Three: The second EMT, at the back of the chair, grasps the uprights of the chair, and leans the chair backwards.

Yes: ❏   Reteach: ❏   Return: ❏   Instructor initials: _____

Step Four: Simultaneously, the two EMTs lift the patient up and proceed to walk forward together.

Yes: ❏   Reteach: ❏   Return: ❏   Instructor initials: _____

Student Name _____ Date _____

Skill 12–12: The Extremity Lift

Equipment Needed:

1. Appropriate PPE

Yes: ❑ Reteach: ❑ Return: ❑ Instructor initials: _____

Step One: The first EMT kneels behind the patient, and helps the patient up to a sitting position. The patient can be rested against the EMTs knee for a moment.

Yes: ❑ Reteach: ❑ Return: ❑ Instructor initials: _____

Step Two: The EMT would then reach under the patient's arms and grasp the patient's wrists, pulling them against the patient's chest tightly.

Yes: ❑ Reteach: ❑ Return: ❑ Instructor initials: _____

Step Three: The second EMT would then crouch between the patient's knees. Reaching down on each side, the EMT would grasp under the patient's knees. (In some cases it may be more convenient to crouch beside the patient's knees and hook arms under the patient's knees.)

Yes: ❑ Reteach: ❑ Return: ❑ Instructor initials: _____

Step Four: Simultaneously, the two EMTs would stand with the patient and walk forward together.

Yes: ❑ Reteach: ❑ Return: ❑ Instructor initials: _____

Student Name _____   Date _____

Skill 12–13: The Direct Lift

Equipment Needed:

1. Appropriate PPE

Yes: ❑   Reteach: ❑   Return: ❑   Instructor initials: _____

Step One: Both of the EMTs stand on one side of the supine patient and then kneel, on the same knee, beside the patient.

Yes: ❑   Reteach: ❑   Return: ❑   Instructor initials: _____

Step Two: The first EMT places one arm under the patient's head and neck, and the other arm under the shoulders. The second EMT places his arms under the patient's lower back and buttocks.

Yes: ❑   Reteach: ❑   Return: ❑   Instructor initials: _____

Step Three: Simultaneously, the two EMTs hoist the patient to their knees. If the patient is being transferred to a stretcher on the other side of the patient, they need only drop the one knee to move forward and over the stretcher.

Yes: ❑   Reteach: ❑   Return: ❑   Instructor initials: _____

Step Four: If the patient is to be carried any distance, the EMTs should roll the patient against their chests and then walk forward together.

Yes: ❑   Reteach: ❑   Return: ❑   Instructor initials: _____

Student Name _____ Date _____

Skill 12–14: Scoop Stretcher

Equipment Needed:

1. Appropriate PPE
2. Orthopedic stretcher

Yes: ❑   Reteach: ❑   Return: ❑   Instructor initials: _____

Step One: The scoop stretcher must be split into its two halves, which must be adjusted to the patient's length.

Yes: ❑   Reteach: ❑   Return: ❑   Instructor initials: _____

Step Two: The patient is then logrolled to one side and the scoop stretcher half placed along the patient's axis. This is repeated with the other side, and the two ends are secured.

Yes: ❑   Reteach: ❑   Return: ❑   Instructor initials: _____

Student Name _____ Date _____

Skill 12–15: End-to-End Stretcher Carry

Equipment Needed:

1. Appropriate PPE
2. Stretcher or litter

Yes: ❏   Reteach: ❏   Return: ❏   Instructor initials: _____

Step One: Each EMT takes a position at each end of the litter. Both EMTs should be facing in the direction of travel. Kneeling down, each EMT grasps a handhold nearest him.

Yes: ❏   Reteach: ❏   Return: ❏   Instructor initials: _____

Step Two: Simultaneously, the EMTs should stand together. If the patient is to be carried any distance, the EMTs should walk forward together.

Yes: ❏   Reteach: ❏   Return: ❏   Instructor initials: _____

Student Name _____ Date _____

Skill 12–16: Diamond Stretcher Carry

Equipment Needed:

1. Appropriate PPE
2. Stretcher or litter

Yes: ❏ Reteach: ❏ Return: ❏ Instructor initials: _____

Step One: An EMT takes a place at each side of the stretcher and one on each end. All EMTs knees should be facing in the direction of travel. Kneeling down, each EMT grasps a handhold nearest him.

Yes: ❏ Reteach: ❏ Return: ❏ Instructor initials: _____

Step Two: Simultaneously, the EMTs should stand. If the patient is to be carried any distance, the EMTs should walk forward together. (Whenever a patient is carried on a stretcher over rough ground, the EMT in charge should chose a diamond carry.)

Yes: ❏ Reteach: ❏ Return: ❏ Instructor initials: _____

Student Name _____ Date _____

Skill 12–17: Four Corners Stretcher Carry

Equipment Needed:

1. Appropriate PPE
2. Stretcher or litter

Yes: ❑   Reteach: ❑   Return: ❑   Instructor initials: _____

Step One: An EMT takes a place at each corner of the stretcher. All EMTs should be facing in the direction of travel. Kneeling down, each EMT grasps a corner of the stretcher.

Yes: ❑   Reteach: ❑   Return: ❑   Instructor initials: _____

Step Two: Simultaneously, the EMTs should stand. If the patient is to be carried any distance, the EMTs should walk forward together.

Yes: ❑   Reteach: ❑   Return: ❑   Instructor initials: _____

Student Name _____ Date _____

Skill 12–18: Use of a Stringer

Equipment Needed:

1. Appropriate PPE
2. Loop of webbing approximately 6 feet long

Yes: ❑   Reteach: ❑   Return: ❑   Instructor initials: _____

Step One: The EMT would place the webbing under the bar, or handhold, and loop it back through itself, in effect creating a half hitch.

Yes: ❑   Reteach: ❑   Return: ❑   Instructor initials: _____

Step Two: The EMT would then kneel next to the stretcher and slip the loop of webbing over his shoulder, being sure that the webbing knot was not on the shoulder.

Yes: ❑   Reteach: ❑   Return: ❑   Instructor initials: _____

Step Three: Then the EMT would slip his opposite hand inside the loop. It may be necessary to shorten the length of the loop by tying a knot in the webbing.

Yes: ❑   Reteach: ❑   Return: ❑   Instructor initials: _____

Step Four: Once standing, the EMT would adjust the loop over his shoulders. One hand should be carrying the stretcher and the other hand should be exerting downward force on the loop, in effect balancing the load.

Yes: ❑   Reteach: ❑   Return: ❑   Instructor initials: _____

Student Name _____ Date _____

Skill 12–19: Caterpillar Pass

Equipment Needed:

1. Appropriate PPE
2. Stretcher or litter

Yes: ❏   Reteach: ❏   Return: ❏   Instructor initials: _____

Step One: Coming to the obstacle, all EMTs stop and turn towards each other.

Yes: ❏   Reteach: ❏   Return: ❏   Instructor initials: _____

Step Two: Two EMTs go around or over the obstacle and take a position across from the litter. The front of the litter is then handed to them across the object.

Yes: ❏   Reteach: ❏   Return: ❏   Instructor initials: _____

Step Three: As the litter is passed forward, the two EMTs in the rear move forward to take position beyond the obstacle. All EMTs remain standing with feet firmly planted as the litter is passed.

Yes: ❏   Reteach: ❏   Return: ❏   Instructor initials: _____

Step Four: Once the litter is beyond and clear of the obstacle, all EMTs turn and face forward. The EMTs may then move forward together as a unit.

Yes: ❏   Reteach: ❏   Return: ❏   Instructor initials: _____

Student Name _____ Date _____

Skill 12–20: Bedroll

Equipment Needed:

1. Appropriate PPE
2. Stretcher, blanket, sheet, pillow, pillowcase

Yes: ❏ Reteach: ❏ Return: ❏ Instructor initials: _____

Step One: The first EMT would lay the blanket centered onto the stretcher, then the sheet on top of that.

Yes: ❏ Reteach: ❏ Return: ❏ Instructor initials: _____

Step Two: The first and second EMT grasp one half of the linen and fold it in half, creating a collar. Repeat with the other side.

Yes: ❏ Reteach: ❏ Return: ❏ Instructor initials: _____

Step Three: To open the bedroll, the EMTs simply grasp the collars and fold the edges.

Yes: ❏ Reteach: ❏ Return: ❏ Instructor initials: _____

Step Four: With the patient lying supine, the EMTs can fold the upper edge over the patient's head, then secure the edge with the lower edge. The pillow should then be placed behind the head, outside the linen.

Yes: ❏ Reteach: ❏ Return: ❏ Instructor initials: _____

Student Name _____ Date _____

Skill 12–21: Carry Transfer

Equipment Needed:

1. Appropriate PPE
2. Two stretchers, gurneys

Yes: ❏   Reteach: ❏   Return: ❏   Instructor initials: _____

Step One: The first stretcher is placed with the patient's head at the foot of the other stretcher at a 90-degree angle.

Yes: ❏   Reteach: ❏   Return: ❏   Instructor initials: _____

Step Two: The two EMTs stand on the side of patient. The first EMT places one arm under the patient's head and neck, and the other arm under the shoulders. The second EMT places his arms under the patient's lower back and buttocks.

Yes: ❏   Reteach: ❏   Return: ❏   Instructor initials: _____

Step Three: Simultaneously, the two EMTs hoist the patient to their chest. Shuffling sideways, the two EMTs move the patient to the awaiting stretcher.

Yes: ❏   Reteach: ❏   Return: ❏   Instructor initials: _____

Step Four: The patient is then gently laid onto the stretcher. The EMT should be sure that all stretcher brakes are engaged before moving the patient.

Yes: ❏   Reteach: ❏   Return: ❏   Instructor initials: _____

97

Student Name _____ Date _____

Skill 12–22: Drawsheet Transfer

Equipment Needed:

1. Appropriate PPE
2. Two stretchers, draw sheet, or bed linen

Yes: ❑   Reteach: ❑   Return: ❑   Instructor initials: _____

Step One: The two stretchers are placed side by side. The EMT should be sure that the stretcher brakes are engaged before moving the patient. Any siderails present will have to be lowered.

Yes: ❑   Reteach: ❑   Return: ❑   Instructor initials: _____

Step Two: Two EMTs are on the one open side of both stretchers. Rolling the edge of the draw sheet or bed linen into a collar, the EMTs grab a firm purchase. (It is a good practice to have the two teams of EMTs pull vigorously against each other to test the strength of the sheet.)

Yes: ❑   Reteach: ❑   Return: ❑   Instructor initials: _____

Step Three: Simultaneously, the four EMTs slide the patient from one stretcher to the other in one fluid motion.

Yes: ❑   Reteach: ❑   Return: ❑   Instructor initials: _____

Step Four: Once the patient is on the new stretcher, the siderails should be replaced.

Yes: ❑   Reteach: ❑   Return: ❑   Instructor initials: _____

CHAPTER 13 SCENE SIZE-UP

This chapter will stress those protective behaviors an EMT should practice while on-scene.

Completion: Complete each of the following sentences using terms from the Key Terms found in Chapter 13 of the textbook.

1. The _____ _____ is the first radio report of the scene conditions.

2. The feeling that there is an increased likelihood of injury is based on a _____ _____ of _____.

3. A device intended to produce death is a(n) _____ _____, while one capable of death or serious harm in certain circumstances is a(n) _____ _____.

4. The _____ divides hazardous areas from nonhazardous areas. A barrier that protects EMTs and permits them to work is a(n) _____ _____.

5. A scene _____ must be done to determine if any hazards are on-scene. Emergency vehicles can then be _____ safely in a specific place.

Identification: For each area of the vehicle, write down information that is relevant to the EMT's damage survey.

1. bumpers _____

2. fenders _____

3. body _____

4. windshield _____

5. passenger compartment _____

6. underneath _____

Identification: Place an X in front of those actions that an EMT should do to assist in vehicle stabilization.

_____ Enter a car sitting on its roof   _____ Close windows

_____ Take the transmission out of drive   _____ Cut seatbelts

_____ Turn off the engine   _____ Engage parking brake

_____ Chock the wheels

True/False: Read each of the following sentences and decide if it is TRUE or FALSE. Place a T or F on the line in front.

1. _____ Upon arrival, the ambulance should be parked right next to the scene to prevent the crew from injuring themselves carrying heavy equipment.

2. _____ The EMT should treat all downed wires as dangerous.

3. _____ The single greatest danger to the EMT at a car crash is leaking fluids.

4. _____ OSHA requires all emergency vehicles to have at least one blue light.

5. _____ The safest place for an ambulance is ahead of the motor vehicle collision.

6. _____ If possible, place the ambulance in the direction of travel to the hospital.

7. _____ Flares are designed to prevent inadvertent ignition of spilled fluids.

8. _____ On a 40 mph straightaway, place the first flare 160 feet from the crash.

9. _____ A starred windshield results from something striking it at a specific point.

10. _____ EMTs provide treatment to multiple patients according to a sorting plan.

Correcting: Rewrite each of the following as a correct statement by replacing or deleting the underlined word or words..

1. On the scene of a major incident, the Safety Officer functions as a member of the <u>operations staff</u>.

2. Stopping the emergency vehicle a safe distance from the scene is called <u>scene survey</u>.

3. Courts have upheld the idea that an EMT <u>cannot refuse</u> to enter a dangerous situation.

4. To place flares on a curve, <u>add two times the radius of the curve</u> to the distance listed on the chart.

Short Answer: Based on each damage descriptor, list the probable point of patient impact.

1. Broken rearview mirror

2. Bent steering wheel

3. Broken dash

4. Seat knocked off pedestal

5. Locked seatbelt

Critical Thinking 1: Read the following scenario. Answer the questions that follow.

Dan and Deborah were called to a gas station following the inadvertent release of dry chemicals from an overhead fire extinguisher system. Once there, they found ten people on the scene, all covered with a white powder. One patron had tripped over the gas can that he was filling, spilling the liquid onto the ground. Another was speaking loudly on a cell phone detailing the reasons she would be late for a meeting.

What scene hazards are present here?

Critical Thinking 2: Read the following scenario. Answer the questions that follow.

Jorge and Marrissa answered a call at the terminus of a high-speed highway. A driver, not paying attention to the END HIGHWAY signs, struck two other cars, resulting in great damage and the leaking of fluids. A police officer has set out flares, but has not closed down the highway.

What scene hazards are present here?

Critical Thinking 3: Read the following scenario. Answer the questions that follow.

Dory and Chris have answered a call at a small out-of-the-way house. While the rest of the area has become suburbanized with new homes and immaculate lawns, this area has remained just as it was sixty years ago; small truck farms with some agricultural animals. There are no sidewalks and no street lights. The home is run down but appears clean. A sign inside the front door reads "Home protected by Smith and Wesson."

What scene hazards are present here?

Student Name _____ Date _____

Skill 13–1: Lighting a Road Flare

Equipment Needed:

1. Road flare
2. Helmet with eye shield
3. Gloves
4. Turnout coat

Yes: ❏   Reteach: ❏   Return: ❏   Instructor initials: _____

Step One: The EMT should first put on minimal eye protection and gloves. It is preferred if the EMT wears a turnout coat as well.

Yes: ❏   Reteach: ❏   Return: ❏   Instructor initials: _____

Step Two: The EMT would then remove the striker from the end of the flare.

Yes: ❏   Reteach: ❏   Return: ❏   Instructor initials: _____

Step Three: The EMT would then briskly strike the striker against the flare's igniter while aiming it away from his body.

Yes: ❏   Reteach: ❏   Return: ❏   Instructor initials: _____

Step Four: The EMT would then keep the lit flare away from his body and place it on the ground.

Yes: ❏   Reteach: ❏   Return: ❏   Instructor initials: _____

Student Name _____ Date _____

Skill 13–2: Vehicle Stabilization

Equipment Needed:

1. Flashlight
2. Turnout gear

Yes: ❏   Reteach: ❏   Return: ❏   Instructor initials: _____

Step One: The first EMT circles the car starting from the driver's side. The EMT advises the patient to sit still for a minute. The EMT checks for vehicle damage.

Yes: ❏   Reteach: ❏   Return: ❏   Instructor initials: _____

Step Two: The second EMT circles the car from the opposite side. The EMT checks for hazards above and underneath the car.

Yes: ❏   Reteach: ❏   Return: ❏   Instructor initials: _____

Step Three: After the second EMT calls "all clear," the first EMT enters the passenger side and takes stabilization of the patient's head.

Yes: ❏   Reteach: ❏   Return: ❏   Instructor initials: _____

Step Four: The first EMT then reaches in and checks to see that the car is in PARK.

Yes: ❏   Reteach: ❏   Return: ❏   Instructor initials: _____

Step Five: The EMT would then confirm the car is turned OFF. The EMT would check for electric locks, windows, and seats first.

Yes: ❏   Reteach: ❏   Return: ❏   Instructor initials: _____

Step Six: The EMT would confirm that the car's emergency brake is engaged.

Yes: ❏   Reteach: ❏   Return: ❏   Instructor initials: _____

CHAPTER 14 INITIAL ASSESSMENT

It is important for the EMT-B to attempt to perform the initial assessment the same way each time. Of course, it will vary slightly depending upon the patient situation, but the order of priorities must always remain the same. This chapter will cover the recommended method of completing an initial assessment.

Identification: Place a check mark in front of those items that should be assessed or found on an initial assessment.

_____ an injured, deformed leg	_____ a stab wound to the chest
_____ vomit in the mouth	_____ absent radial pulse
_____ history of a heart attack	_____ allergy to penicillin
_____ crepitus over the neck and chest	_____ snoring respirations
_____ a bone deformed in the arm	_____ blood-soaked jeans
_____ gives a complete medical history	_____ breakfast last eaten
_____ use of cocaine	_____ tenderness of chest wall

Identification: Decide if each patient is alert, verbal, responsive to pain, or unresponsive. Place the correct letter, A, V, P, or U on the line before each description.

1. _____ The patient asks appropriate questions.

2. _____ There is no movement at all when a woman's skin is pinched.

3. _____ A man moans "uh huh" if spoken to loudly.

4. _____ The patient only moves if pressure is applied to his fingernail.

5. _____ A child watches where Mom and Dad go.

6. _____ A woman speaks rapidly to the EMT-B in a foreign language.

7. _____ The patient appears to go to sleep when the EMT-B stops talking.

8. _____ A child opens his eyes when spoken to in a loud voice.

9. _____ A patient opens his eyes only when the shoulder is pinched.

Sorting: Place the following descriptions under the correct heading of patent airway or nonpatent airway.

snoring	broken teeth in mouth	very bloody nose
speaking clearly	stridor	quiet breathing
drooling	vomitus	good chest rise
unresponsive	infant unable to cry	alert and oriented

Patent   **Nonpatent**

True or False: Read each statement and decide if it is TRUE or FALSE. Place T or F on line before each statement.

1. _____ Breathing is checked after the pulse.

2. _____ To adequately check breathing, look, listen, and feel.

3. _____ An adequate respiratory rate for an adult is between 10 and 28 breaths per minute.

4. _____ Chest injuries may impair breathing adequacy.

5. _____ Open chest wounds impede adequate lung expansion.

6. _____ Wheezing may indicate a partial airway obstruction.

7. _____ Subcutaneous air feels like a sponge.

8. _____ Check for a pulse on an infant at the radius.

9. _____ When checking a pulse in a hypothermic patient, count for one full minute.

10. _____ All bleeding should be immediately controlled.

11. _____ Capillary refill is a good indicator of perfusion in a 2-year-old.

Definitions: Define the following terms.

1. alert _____

2. crepitus _____

3. sternal rub _____

4. flail chest _____

5. paradoxical motion _____

6. AVPU _____

7. ABCs _____

8. unresponsive _____

Short Answer: Read each question. Think about the information presented in your text, and then answer each question with one or two sentences.

1. What does the "look test" tell the EMT?

2. During the B step of the initial assessment, the EMT finds that the patient is breathing. What other information must he obtain before he moves on in his assessment?

3. What type(s) of bleeding must be controlled during the initial assessment?

Determining priority: Read each patient presentation and determine if the patient is high or low priority. Place the word on the line in front of each presentation.

_____ Looks ill

_____ Has a swollen deformed arm

_____ Is complaining of some dizziness

_____ Verbally responds but doesn't follow commands

_____ Back pain after a motor vehicle collision

_____ Respiratory rate 34 and shallow

_____ Excessive bleeding from a leg wound

_____ Anxious, rapid breathing and pulse

_____ Normal childbirth

Critical Thinking 1: Read the scenario. Answer the questions that follow.

Jeff and Makenzi were called to the dorm room of a young male patient who would not wake up. His buddies said he had spent the night cramming for an exam and when they went to get him today, they couldn't get him to wake up.

The EMT-Bs found a young man lying supine on the floor of his dorm room. His skin was very pale and he didn't answer when his name was called.

1. Is there a potentially life-threatening condition present? If so, what is it?

2. Based on the limited information available, what should the EMT-Bs anticipate with regard to the airway?

3. What priority would you assign to this patient?

Critical Thinking 2: Read the scenario. Answer the questions that follow.

Fran and Eric answered a call to the local nursing home for a patient not feeling well. Upon their arrival, they found Mr. Edgars sitting at the end of his bed. He told the EMT-Bs that his stomach had been upset for two days and he didn't feel much like eating. He also said he hadn't vomited, just that he felt "yecchy."

1. Is there a potentially life-threatening condition present? If so, what is it?

2. Based on the limited information available, what do the EMT-Bs know about Mr. Edgars airway?

3. What priority would you assign to this patient?

Critical Thinking 3: Read the scenario. Answer the questions that follow.

Dean and Donny were dispatched to a woman ready to give birth. Upon their arrival, they found Mrs. Green lying on her couch. She looked pale and sweaty. There was an excessive amount of blood present on her clothing and she complained of unbearable pain.

1. Is there a potentially life-threatening condition present? If so, what is it?

2. Based on the limited information available, what should the EMT-Bs anticipate with regard to perfusion?

3. What priority would you assign to this patient?

Student Name _____ Date _____

Skill 14–1: Initial Assessment

Purpose: To obtain a baseline examination for assessment and comparison, as well as detection and treatment of life-threatening injuries.

Standard Precautions:
- Hand washing
- Gloves

Equipment Needed:

1. Stethoscope
2. Scissors

Yes: ❑   Reteach: ❑   Return: ❑   Instructor initials: _____

Step One: The EMT surveys the scene for safety hazards as well as any potential mechanism of injury. Needed personal protective equipment would be donned now.

Yes: ❑   Reteach: ❑   Return: ❑   Instructor initials: _____

Step Two: The EMT forms a general impression of the scene; decideing, for example, whether it was trauma or medical.

Yes: ❑   Reteach: ❑   Return: ❑   Instructor initials: _____

Step Three: The EMT next determines mental status on the AVPU Scale. If the scene was trauma, another EMT immediately takes head stabilization first.

Yes: ❑   Reteach: ❑   Return: ❑   Instructor initials: _____

Step Four: The EMT assesses and manages the airway, as needed.

Yes: ❑   Reteach: ❑   Return: ❑   Instructor initials: _____

Step Five: Next, the EMT assesses and manages breathing.

Yes: ❑   Reteach: ❑   Return: ❑   Instructor initials: _____

Step Six: Finally, the EMT assesses and manages circulation. If the patient is high priority, transportation should be initiated immediately.

Yes: ❑   Reteach: ❑   Return: ❑   Instructor initials: _____

CHAPTER 15   FOCUSED HISTORY AND PHYSICAL EXAMINATION OF THE TRAUMA PATIENT

Once the initial assessment is complete and no life threats found, the EMT-B will complete the focused history and physical exam.

Word Scramble: Unscramble the following terms.

1. nobarsia   _____

2. nubr   _____

3. ustnncooi   _____

4. ytorfmied   _____

5. gradguin   _____

6. craatilnoe   _____

7. uuptcner   _____

8. liwsnelg   _____

9. trened   _____

10. tiprecsu   _____

True or False: Read each statement and decide if it is TRUE or FALSE. Place T or F on line before each statement.

1. _____   It is easy to determine if a patient has a medical or a trauma problem.

2. _____   All patients are trauma until proven otherwise.

3. _____   The medical history is gathered after the trauma physical exam.

4. _____   The rapid trauma exam is used to find injuries not initially evident.

5. _____   In minor trauma, the EMT-B performs a focused trauma exam.

6. _____   All unconscious patients should have a rapid trauma exam.

7. _____   Gruesome bone injuries require immediate attention.

8. _____   All trauma patients need spinal immobilization.

9. _____   The initial assessment is performed only once.

10. _____   A rapid trauma exam begins at the head and progresses to the feet.

Listing: List six principles for conducting a physical exam.

1. _____

2. _____

3. _____

4. _____

5. _____

6. _____

Identification: Place a check mark in front of the serious trauma by mechanisms.

_____ Vehicle rollover with unrestrained patient

_____ Fall of 10 feet

_____ Death of another occupant in the vehicle

_____ Farm trauma

_____ Vehicle/pedestrian accident

_____ Twenty inches of front-end damage

_____ Ejection

_____ Motorcycle accident

_____ Crash speed of 20 mph or greater

Ordering: Put the steps for completing a rapid trauma exam in order by placing the numeral 1 before the first step, 2 before the second, and so on.

_____ Obtain baseline vitals signs

_____ Document

_____ Size-up/scene safety

_____ Obtain a SAMPLE history

_____ Complete an initial assessment, including spinal precautions

_____ Consider ALS

_____ Complete a rapid trauma assessment

Completion: Write out the word suggested by each letter of the acronym. Explain what each word means.

D

C

A

P

B

T

L

S

What does this acronym remind the EMT-B to do?

Short Answer 1: Read the scenario and answer the questions that follow.

A teenager trips on a high curb and injures his right ankle. There is no fall, and no loss of consciousness.

1. Would this be considered major or minor trauma according to the table of serious mechanisms?

2. From your textbook, list the exams that will be performed.

Short Answer 2: Read the scenario and answer the questions that follow.

A young man is involved in a rollover accident on the interstate.

1. Would this be considered major or minor trauma according to the table of serious mechanisms?

2. From your textbook, list the exams that will be performed.

Short Answer 3: Read the scenario and answer the questions that follow.

A roofer falls from a church steeple.

1. Would this be considered major or minor trauma according to the table of serious mechanisms?

2. From your textbook, list the exams that will be performed.

Short Answer 4: Read the scenario and answer the questions that follow.

A woman is struck by the side of a car just as the car is leaving a stoplight.

1. Would this be considered major or minor trauma according to the table of serious mechanisms?

2. From your textbook, list the exams that will be performed.

Short Answer 5: Read the scenario and answer the questions that follow.

A skateboarder falls down six steps at the public library. There is no loss of consciousness.

1. Would this be considered major or minor trauma according to the table of serious mechanisms?

2. From your textbook, list the exams that will be performed.

Student Name _____ Date _____

Skill 15–1: Rapid Trauma Assessment

Purpose: To assess for other non-life-threatening injuries of the major trauma patient.

Standard Precautions:
- Hand washing
- Gloves

Equipment Needed:

1. Penlight
2. Stethoscope
3. Cervical collars
4. Blood pressure cuff
5. Scissors

Yes: ❏   Reteach: ❏   Return: ❏   Instructor initials: _____

Step One: After completing an appropriate scene size-up and initial assessment, the EMT performs a rapid trauma assessment on the trauma patient with a significant mechanism of injury. Manual head stabilization is maintained for the duration of the rapid trauma assessment.

Yes: ❏   Reteach: ❏   Return: ❏   Instructor initials: _____

Step Two: The EMT should consider a request for ALS backup and determine the transport priority. Transport begins.

Yes: ❏   Reteach: ❏   Return: ❏   Instructor initials: _____

Step Three: The EMT next assesses the head by careful inspection and palpation for signs of injury. Deformities, contusions, abrasions, punctures/penetrations, burns, tenderness, lacerations, or swelling should be noted. Moving in a methodical fashion, the EMT next inspects and palpates the neck.

Yes: ❏   Reteach: ❏   Return: ❏   Instructor initials: _____

Step Four: The EMT next looks, listens, and feels the chest to assess for presence of any signs of injury. Breath sounds are carefully assessed at the apices and bases. Presence and equality of air movement is noted.

Yes: ❏   Reteach: ❏   Return: ❏   Instructor initials: _____

Step Five: The abdominal assessment includes looking and feeling for any signs of injury. The pelvis is visually inspected, then gently compressed downward and inward in order to find any signs of injury.

Yes: ❏   Reteach: ❏   Return: ❏   Instructor initials: _____

(continues)

Skill 15–1: Continued

Step Six: After rolling the patient to the side using a logroll technique, maintaining spinal immobilization, the EMT inspects and palpates the back and buttocks to find signs of injury.

Yes: ❑   Reteach: ❑   Return: ❑   Instructor initials: _____

Step Seven: After completing the rapid trauma assessment, a complete baseline set of vital signs must be taken.

Yes: ❑   Reteach: ❑   Return: ❑   Instructor initials: _____

Step Eight: A SAMPLE history is elicited.

Yes: ❑   Reteach: ❑   Return: ❑   Instructor initials: _____

Student Name _____ Date _____

Skill 15–2: Focused Trauma Assessment

Purpose: To obtain a baseline physical examination for assessment and comparison of the minor trauma patient.

Standard Precautions:
- Hand washing
- Gloves
- Goggles
- Gown

Equipment Needed:

1. Stethoscope
2. Blood pressure cuff
3. Assortment of cervical collars

Yes: ❑   Reteach: ❑   Return: ❑   Instructor initials: _____

Step One: The EMT considers the mechanism of injury. Depending on the mechanism of injury, the EMT decides whether to perform a rapid trauma assessment or a focused physical examination.

Yes: ❑   Reteach: ❑   Return: ❑   Instructor initials: _____

Step Two: The EMT next determines the chief complaint.

Yes: ❑   Reteach: ❑   Return: ❑   Instructor initials: _____

Step Three: The EMT performs a focused examination specific to the injury.

Yes: ❑   Reteach: ❑   Return: ❑   Instructor initials: _____

Step Four: The EMT then obtains baseline vital signs.

Yes: ❑   Reteach: ❑   Return: ❑   Instructor initials: _____

Step Five: The EMT completes the assessment with a SAMPLE history.

Yes: ❑   Reteach: ❑   Return: ❑   Instructor initials: _____

CHAPTER 16 DETAILED PHYSICAL EXAMINATION

The detailed physical exam is a patient-specific and injury-specific examination. It is performed on patients who have significant injuries or a significant mechanism of injury.

Matching: Match word or phrase with its definition. Place the letter of the correct definition on the line in front of the term.

1. _____ aniscoria
2. _____ Battle's sign
3. _____ cerebrospinal fluid
4. _____ halo test
5. _____ hyphema
6. _____ PERRL
7. _____ raccoon eyes
8. _____ seat belt sign
9. _____ PMS
10. _____ urinary incontinence

a. bruising behind the ears
b. a ring of CSF around blood
c. description of normal pupils
d. a red mark left by a car restraint device
e. pulses, motor, sensory
f. blood in the anterior chamber of the eye
g. fluid that bathes the spinal cord and brain
h. loss of control of the bladder
i. unequal pupils
j. bruising around the eyes

True or False: Read each statement and decide if it is TRUE or FALSE. Place T or F on line before each statement.

1. _____ Compression/flexion of the pelvis is not indicated if a pelvic injury is already suspected.
2. _____ The detailed physical exam is focused on the complaint only.
3. _____ The detailed physical exam is performed on patients with serious injuries.
4. _____ Use DCAPBTLS as the mnemonic for the detailed physical exam.
5. _____ Apply direct pressure to stop the flow of CSF from the nose or ears.
6. _____ In the halo test, blood will spread out and around the CSF.
7. _____ Bruising behind the ears may indicate a fracture at the base of the skull.
8. _____ Bruising around the eyes is indicative of a temporal skull fracture.
9. _____ Unequal pupils always indicate a head injury.
10. _____ Loose dentures should be removed.

Ordering: Place a 1 before the action that should be completed first, a 2 in front of the next action, and so on.

_____ Rapid trauma exam

_____ First impression

_____ Scene survey/size-up

_____ Detailed exam

_____ Initial exam

Listing: List the specific things that should be assessed in each region.

skull   _____

ears   _____

eyes   _____

face   _____

nose   _____

mouth   _____

neck   _____

chest   _____

abdomen   _____

extremities _____

Critical Thinking 1: Read the scenario and then answer the questions that follow.

Tom and Howard answered to a call at a construction site. A construction worker had fallen 10 feet from scaffolding to a sandy surface. First responders indicated that the worker had probably suffered a head injury.

1. What injuries should the EMTs discover in the initial exam?

2. What injuries should the EMTs discover in the detailed physical exam that would lead to the conclusion of a head injury?

Critical Thinking 2: Georgette and Christopher were on their way to quarters when they came upon a motor vehicle collision. The primary ambulance crew had triaged patients, and Georgette and Chris were assigned to care for a 60-year-old man who was a restrained passenger in a vehicle that was struck head on. Mr. Smith complained of feeling "shaken" but otherwise unhurt. The car suffered extensive front-end damage. The initial assessment showed "no life threats." Rapid trauma exam showed a reddened area across the abdomen and right shoulder. No other injuries were noted. While the EMTs were completing the detailed exam, the patient complained that he felt anxious and thirsty and that his heart was racing.

1. What further injuries can be expected on the detailed physical exam?

2. What problem might explain the increased heart rate, change in mental status, and injuries noted on the detailed exam?

Student Name _____ Date _____

Skill 16–1: Detailed Physical Examination

Purpose: To obtain a more thorough physical examination of injuries to a trauma patient, usually performed en route to the hospital.

Standard Precautions:
- Hand washing
- Gloves
- Goggles
- Gown

Equipment Needed:

1. Penlight
2. Stethoscope
3. Blood pressure cuff
4. Scissors

Yes: ❏   Reteach: ❏   Return: ❏   Instructor initials: _____

Step One: Start at the top of the head and assess the scalp and the face for DCAP-BTLS.

Yes: ❏   Reteach: ❏   Return: ❏   Instructor initials: _____

Step Two: Next, assess the ears, nose, and throat, noting any bleeding or drainage of fluids, as well as jugular venous distention or displacement of the trachea.

Yes: ❏   Reteach: ❏   Return: ❏   Instructor initials: _____

Step Three: Then, proceed to looking, listening, and feeling the chest wall for injury, including crepitus and paradoxical motion.

Yes: ❏   Reteach: ❏   Return: ❏   Instructor initials: _____

Step Four: Turning next to the abdomen and the pelvis, assess for DCAP-BTLS. Assessment of the pelvis should include gentle pressure inward on the hips to check for a hip fracture.

Yes: ❏   Reteach: ❏   Return: ❏   Instructor initials: _____

Step Five: Then, assess the extremities for pulses, movement, and sensation, as well as DCAP-BTLS.

Yes: ❏   Reteach: ❏   Return: ❏   Instructor initials: _____

(continues)

Skill 16–1: Continued

Step Six: After checking as much of the posterior as possible, obtain another set of vital signs.

Yes: ❏   Reteach: ❏   Return: ❏   Instructor initials: _____

117

CHAPTER 17 FOCUSED HISTORY AND PHYSICAL FOR THE MEDICAL PATIENT

The priorities of a patient suffering from a medical illness become somewhat different than the patient suffering from a trauma. These priorities change based upon whether the medical patient is awake and responsive or unresponsive.

Sorting: Place the information into its correct category.

headache	asthma attack 1 week ago	eczema
hives with penicillin	wheezing after eating nuts	ate breakfast
Ventolin q6 hours	aspirin daily	cleaning with bleach
asthma	Theodur QID	shortness of breath

S   A   M   P   L   E

Ordering: Place in order of completion for a responsive medical patient.

_____ Ongoing assessment

_____ Chief complaint

_____ SAMPLE

_____ Baseline vital signs

_____ OPQRST

_____ Initial assessment

_____ Treat and transport

_____ Focused physical exam

Ordering: Place in order of completion for an unresponsive medical patient.

_____ SAMPLE history

_____ Initial assessment

_____ Treat and transport

_____ Baseline vital signs

_____ Rapid physical exam

_____ Ongoing assessment

Short Answer: For each patient, decide which assessment format you will use.

1. _____ Unconscious, lying in bed

2. _____ Awake, crying, cut hand on glass

3. _____ Unconscious at base of ladder

4. _____ Walked into station complaining of a headache

5. _____ Superficial stab wound to thigh

6. _____ Gunshot wound to the chest

7. _____ Severe cough and fever

8. _____ Not responding after eating cookies

9. _____ Abdominal pain after car crash

10. _____ Abdominal pain and vomiting after dinner

Definitions: Write the definition of each word or term in the space provided.

1. chief complaint _____

2. focused physical exam _____

3. medic alert bracelet _____

4. ongoing assessment _____

5. on-line medical control _____

6. OPQRST _____

7. SAMPLE _____

8. vial of life _____

True or False: Read each statement and decide if it is TRUE or FALSE. Place T or F on line before each statement.

1. _____ The history of the present illness in a medical patient is the equivalent of the mechanism of injury for the trauma patient.

2. _____ The chief complaint is determined by the EMT after the focused exam is completed.

3. _____ The history should guide the EMT in focusing the physical exam.

4. _____ Abnormal vital signs should prompt the EMT to initiate immediate transport.

5. _____ The rapid physical exam for the medical patient is conducted in the same way as for the trauma patient.

6. _____ Transport should always be initiated before the rapid trauma exam.

7. _____ If an EMT has a question about providing a treatment, he should arrange an ALS intercept.

8. _____ Contact with the receiving facility should include the nature of the patient's problem.

9. _____ All medical patients are managed in the same way.

Critical Thinking 1: Read the scenario and answer the questions following it.

Steve and Donna were assessing an unresponsive patient found in bed by family members.

1. Name at least three ways to obtain information on this patient.

2. When would transport be initiated for this patient?

Critical Thinking 2: Read the scenario and answer the questions following it.

Dana and Greg were attending to Mrs. Fleming, who called complaining of a headache. As the EMTs were obtaining the SAMPLE history, Mrs. Fleming also told them about an upset stomach, pain in both legs, dizziness, and lack of appetite.

1. What is the chief complaint?

Student Name _____ Date _____

Skill 17–1: Focused Medical Assessment—Responsive Patient

Purpose: To obtain a baseline examination of the responsive medical patient.

Standard Precautions:
- Hand washing
- Gloves

Equipment Needed:

1. Penlight
2. Stethoscope
3. Blood pressure cuff
4. Scissors

Yes: ❏   Reteach: ❏   Return: ❏   Instructor initials: _____

Step One: Obtain a chief complaint and a history of the present illness, using the OPQRST format when appropriate.

Yes: ❏   Reteach: ❏   Return: ❏   Instructor initials: _____

Step Two: After obtaining the history of the present illness, take the patient's SAMPLE history.

Yes: ❏   Reteach: ❏   Return: ❏   Instructor initials: _____

Step Three: On the basis of the patient's chief complaint, perform a focused physical examination of the affected area. After the physical examination, obtain a baseline set of vital signs.

Yes: ❏   Reteach: ❏   Return: ❏   Instructor initials: _____

Step Four: It may be necessary to assist the patient with his medications, or transport the patient to the hospital. An ongoing assessment should be continued en route to the hospital.

Yes: ❏   Reteach: ❏   Return: ❏   Instructor initials: _____

Student Name _____   Date _____

Skill 17–2: Rapid Medical Examination—Unresponsive Patient

Purpose: To obtain a baseline examination of the unresponsive medical patient.

Standard Precautions:
• Hand washing
• Gloves

Equipment Needed:

1. Penlight
2. Stethoscope
3. Blood pressure cuff
4. Scissors

Yes: ❏   Reteach: ❏   Return: ❏   Instructor initials: _____

Step One: Quickly perform an initial assessment.

Yes: ❏   Reteach: ❏   Return: ❏   Instructor initials: _____

Step Two: Proceed to a rapid physical examination of the patient.

Yes: ❏   Reteach: ❏   Return: ❏   Instructor initials: _____

Step Three: As soon as is practical, a baseline set of vital signs is obtained as well.

Yes: ❏   Reteach: ❏   Return: ❏   Instructor initials: _____

Step Four: Bystanders or family members should be questioned about the patient's illness and past medical history.

Yes: ❏   Reteach: ❏   Return: ❏   Instructor initials: _____

Step Five: Transport the patient as soon as possible.

Yes: ❏   Reteach: ❏   Return: ❏   Instructor initials: _____

Step Six: En route to the hospital, contact medical control and consider meeting with ALS.

Yes: ❏   Reteach: ❏   Return: ❏   Instructor initials: _____

CHAPTER 18 THE ONGOING ASSESSMENT

The EMT is responsible for observing and caring for the patient until arrival at the hospital, where care will be turned over to the hospital staff.

Short Answer: From your reading, answer the following questions.

1. State two reasons for performing the ongoing assessment.

2. When is the ongoing assessment conducted?

Identification: Place an X next to those items evaluated in the ongoing assessment.

_____ mental status	_____ history
_____ airway	_____ pulses
_____ SAMPLE	_____ effectiveness of meds
_____ baseline vital signs	_____ home safety
_____ breathing	_____ abrasions to forearms
_____ empty oxygen tank	_____ bleeding
_____ pulse oximetry	_____ pulse, respirations, BP
_____ distal pulses	

Critical Thinking: Locate the trends in each scenario, and then indicate whether the patient's condition (priority) has changed.

1. Ongoing assessment shows that the pulse rate has increased by 20 beats per minute, and the patient is now extremely anxious.

2. The respiratory rate has dropped from 28 breaths per minute to 20 breaths per minute. The patient can now say five words per breath as opposed to two words per breath.

3. The patient had been answering questions appropriately. Now he is increasingly sleepy and gives only one-word answers.

Student Name _____ Date _____

Skill 18–1: Ongoing Assessment

Purpose: To continue to monitor the patient for assessment and comparison to baseline examinations.

Standard Precautions:
- Hand washing
- Gloves

Equipment Needed:

1. Penlight
2. Stethoscope
3. Blood pressure cuff

Yes: ❑   Reteach: ❑   Return: ❑   Instructor initials: _____

Step One: While en route to the hospital, repeat the initial assessment, reassessing the patient's mental status using the AVPU scale, and monitoring the airway.

Yes: ❑   Reteach: ❑   Return: ❑   Instructor initials: _____

Step Two: The patient's breathing must be reassessed for rate and quality, and lung sounds must be monitored.

Yes: ❑   Reteach: ❑   Return: ❑   Instructor initials: _____

Step Three: Reassess the patient's circulatory status, including skin temperature, and note any additional bleeding.

Yes: ❑   Reteach: ❑   Return: ❑   Instructor initials: _____

Step Four: After mentally reviewing the patient's priorities, reassess vital signs and repeat a physical examination as needed.

Yes: ❑   Reteach: ❑   Return: ❑   Instructor initials: _____

Step Five: Recheck the interventions, such as oxygen tank pressures.

Yes: ❑   Reteach: ❑   Return: ❑   Instructor initials: _____

CHAPTER 19 RADIO

EMTs need a rudimentary understanding of communication systems and how to operate them. These systems are a part of the daily life of an EMT.

Definitions: Write the definition of the following terms.

1. base station _____

2. communications center _____

3. communications specialist _____

4. med channel _____

5. tactical channel _____

6. trunked line _____

Matching: Match word or words with the definition. Place the letter of the correct definition on the line in front of the term.

1. _____ affirmative
2. _____ digital technology
3. _____ FM radio
4. _____ echo technique

5. _____ negative
6. _____ channel crowding
7. _____ scanner
8. _____ UHF
9. _____ special codes
10. _____ hailing frequency
11. _____ VHF
12. _____ repeater
13. _____ megahertz
14. _____ frequency
15. _____ simplex

a. multiple users on one frequency
b. radio code, replacing words
c. channel used to call a specific agency or hospital
d. a radio that can transmit or receive but not at the same time
e. a wave speed measurement
f. very high frequency
g. term meaning "yes"
h. radio that alters the speed of a wave
i. picks up a signal and boosts it
j. also known as a channel
k. ultra high frequency
l. a device permitting the public to listen to EMS channels
m. term meaning "no"
n. repetition to confirm what was said
o. conversion into digitally coded signals

Listing: List the six roles of a communications specialist.

1.

2.

3.

4.

5.

6.

Identification: Place the name of the radio system component on the line before each description.

1. _____ Wireless electronic device permitting transmission of messages to radio receivers

2. _____ Large powerful radio located at a stationary site

3. _____ Radio located inside a vehicle

4. _____ Receiver that picks up the signal and boosts it

5. _____ Handheld radio

6. _____ Radio that either receives or transmits, but not both at same time

7. _____ Radio similar in nature to a phone

Sorting: Read the information below. If the information should be part of an alert report, mark A. If it is part of a consultation report, mark C. If it is part of both reports, mark B.

_____ unit identifier   _____ age/gender

_____ ETA   _____ chief complaint

_____ mental status   _____ vital signs

_____ treatments in progress   _____ SAMPLE

_____ exam findings   _____ changes after treatments

Short Answer: Answer the following questions from your reading.

1. How do communications specialists protect the public during an EMS call?

2. Name three ways in which communications specialists reduce injury or death of patients who call for EMS assistance.

3. Why are communications specialists called the "first first responders"?

4. Describe the role of the FCC in EMS communications.

Critical Thinking: Read the following scenario and write both an alert report and a consultation report for each.

ARS unit 1, a BLS response vehicle, arrived at the scene of a 70-year-old woman living in a retirement home. Her neighbors reported that she "wasn't acting herself" that day. The woman just said her head hurt a lot. She had participated in card games the evening before and seemed OK. It was only today that anyone noticed a change. Medicines located on the kitchen counter included pills for high blood pressure, eye drops for glaucoma, and a daily aspirin.

The woman was awake, but couldn't seem to get simple answers straight. She also kept complaining of her headache. Initial and focused exams showed no signs of bleeding or injury. Lung sounds were clear. Respirations were 16 per minute and non-labored. Her pulse was strong at the wrist and 64 per minute and regular. BP was 198/98. There was a noticeable droop to her mouth as she tried to smile, and her left-hand grasp was much weaker than the right.

The EMTs placed her onto the stretcher, began high-flow oxygen, and requested an ALS intercept. They hoped to meet up with the ALS within 10 minutes. It would take them 20 minutes to arrive at the hospital.

CHAPTER 20 REPORT

Giving a patient report offers two health care professionals an opportunity to focus on one patient and exchange observations, records, and physical findings.

Definitions: Give an example of each of the following terms.

abandonment _____

confidentiality _____

repetitive persistence _____

verbal report _____

Listing: List the three rights of effective interpersonal communications.

1.

2.

3.

Critical Thinking 1: Read the scenario and answer the statements following it.

Jeff and Suzanne arrived at the ED with Mr. Hayes. Jeff said he would give report to a nurse so the ambulance could get back into service. Jeff approached the first person in white that he saw and began to give a quick report on Mr. Hayes. The woman told Jeff that she was not the person to talk to, that he should try the nurse in Room 23.

1. Give at least three reasons why the woman would not accept the report from Jeff.

2. Suggest two ways in which Jeff could have discovered the reasons for the woman to direct him elsewhere.

Critical Thinking 2: Read the scenario and answer the statement following it.

Jeff had found the correct nurse to give report to, but felt that she was not listening to him.

1. Suggest at least two ways in which Jeff could assure himself that the nurse was listening to the report.

Critical Thinking 3: Read the scenario and answer the statements following it.

While Jeff was giving the report, the nurse indicated that she would prefer for the patient to answer the questions.

1. Suggest two reasons that the nurse would want to obtain information from the patient directly.

2. List those pieces of information that should have been provided by the EMT to the nurse.

CHAPTER 21 RECORD

An EMT, as a part of the medical team, is held to the same documentation standards as any other health care provider.

True or False: Read each statement and decide if it is TRUE or FALSE. Place T or F on the line before each statement.

1. _____ The chief complaint is the basis for care.

2. _____ Continuous quality improvement is an ongoing process.

3. _____ Persons who are required by law to report certain situations are mandated reporters.

4. _____ The minimum data set describes what happened to create an injury.

5. _____ The patient care report is a hospital-based form.

6. _____ The patient will sign a special incident report if he refuses care or transport.

7. _____ The agency medical director may review a sentinel PCR.

8. _____ A triage tag is used by the triage nurse to make room assignments.

Fill in the Blank: Complete each sentence with one of the Key Terms found in Chapter 21 of the textbook.

1. Written testimony is made on a(n)_____.

2. Information obtained by direct observation or measurement is _____ in nature.

3. The "P" in SOAP stands for _____.

4. A(n) _____ observation is something that the EMT cannot directly see or measure.

5. A(n) _____ observation is something that can be measured.

6. The chief complaint would be an example of _____ information.

7. "The patient fell from the ladder" is an example of the _____ _____ _____.

8. The document that an EMT would use to describe a stretcher malfunction is the _____ _____ _____.

Listing: List four functions of the PCR.

1.

2.

3.

4.

Short Answer: Answer each of the following from your reading.

1. Describe the differences between an open format PCR and a closed format PCR.

2. When is a closed format especially useful?

3. When is an open format useful?

Critical Thinking: Read the following scenario. Then document the patient encounter using both SOAP and CHEATED.

XYZ Ambulance Service was sent to the scene of a car that had collided into a tree. Witnesses reported that the car did not try to stop. There were no skid marks noted on the road. The speed limit in the area was 40 mph. The only occupant of the car was the driver, Mr. Kardis. The first responders stated that they removed his seat belt when beginning their assessment. Mr. Kardis complained that it hurt to breathe. He said that his cell phone rang, and when he went to answer it, he became distracted. The EMTs noted that the car was stable, there were no overhanging branches, and the windshield was intact. Mr. Kardis denied losing consciousness. He was speaking clearly, but only at 2–3 words per breath. His face was drawn tight and he grimaced each time he took a breath. The steering wheel was intact, but the airbag had deployed. Mr. Kardis was breathing 26 times per minute. His pulse rate was 100, and the first responders reported a blood pressure of 116/76. There was no evidence of any broken bones or obvious bleeding. Lung sounds were clear, although it hurt when the stethoscope was placed on the right side of the ribs. Mr. Kardis was started on 15 lpm of oxygen by NRB mask. His C-spine was protected. Collar was applied and a short spine device was used to remove him to a long spine board. He had good extremity pulses, and could feel and move all extremities before and after the move. He told the EMTs that he was allergic to penicillin, took a pill for his high blood pressure, and had a hernia operation 3 years ago. He had just finished lunch, and was on his way back to work when the accident occurred.

CHAPTER 22 PHARMACOLOGY FOR THE STREET

The study of medications and their interactions is called pharmacology. The EMT-B is responsible for basic pharmacology related to commonly encountered medicines.

Identification: Read the definitions. Write the correct word or terms on the line.

1. _____ A specific circumstance in which not to give a drug

2. _____ Medications that open narrowed airways

3. _____ Instructions to guide treatment decisions

4. _____ Effects of a medication

5. _____ Amount of the medication given

6. _____ Last date that the drug is guaranteed to be effective

7. _____ Physician input into writing protocols

8. _____ An unintended drug effect

9. _____ Reason for giving a medication

10. _____ Protocols that can be followed without speaking with a physician

Identification: Place a check mark in front of each word or phrase that is a generic name for a drug.

____ ventolin   ____ pseudoephedrine   ____ acetaminophen

____ ibuprofen   ____ sudafed   ____ motrin

____ advil   ____ albuterol   ____ tylenol

True or False: Read each statement and decide if it is TRUE or FALSE. Place T or F on line before each statement.

1. _____ Give oxygen based on the oxygen saturation reading.

2. _____ For suspected low blood sugar in an awake patient, give instaglucose.

3. _____ Administer activated charcoal to an unconscious poisoned patient.

4. _____ Assist a patient in respiratory distress to use his albuterol inhaler.

5. _____ Assist a hypotensive patient with chest pain to take a nitro tab.

6. _____ Administer a friend's EpiPen to a patient stung by a bee.

7. _____ Assist a child in holding the oxygen mask.

8. _____ Give activated charcoal to a child who ate Tylenol tabs yesterday.

Naming: For each description, write the name of the drug form.

1. _____ A powder compressed into a shape

2. _____ A temperature-sensitive, thick fluid that can be administered and absorbed from the mouth

3. _____ A powder that floats in a liquid and is more palatable

4. _____ A powder that floats on air and is inhaled into the lungs

5. _____ Oxygen is the primary medicinal one

Naming: For each description, write the correct route of administration.

1. _____ Inside the veins of the body

2. _____ Inside the mouth

3. _____ Space just under the skin

4. _____ Into the deep muscle

5. _____ Creating a mist to be inhaled

6. _____ Under the tongue

Listing: List the five rights of drug administration.

1. _____

2. _____

3. _____

4. _____

5. _____

Fill in the Blank: Read the following paragraph on documentation and complete the missing words.

The EMT-B must _____ the patient and include physical and historical information on the patient care record. List the exact _____ of the drug, the _____, or how much was given, and the _____, or the way it was given. Within 5 minutes of giving the medication, a _____ of the patient should be done and findings from this should be included on the patient care record. Be sure to evaluate the signs or symptoms that led to the use of the medication originally.

Completion: Complete the following table.

Drug indications	Contraindications	Actions	Side effects	Dose/route
charcoal				
oral glucose				
oxygen				
albuterol				
nitroglycerin				
epinephrine				

Critical Thinking 1: Read the scenario. Determine which drug the patient should have, give at least one reason for the patient to have that drug, and list the things that must be reassessed after giving the drug.

Rhonda and Geoff were dispatched to the home of an elderly man who was having difficulty breathing. When they arrived, they found him sitting straight upright in a chair. He could only say one word per breath. He admitted that he was afraid to move because he wouldn't be able to get enough air. Physical exam showed wheezing in both lungs, use of accessory muscles for breathing, a respiratory rate of 24 and labored, a pulse of 88 and regular, and a blood pressure of 136/88. The difficulty breathing began that day when the man had been outside working in his garden during a spell of hot humid weather. His past medical history included asthma, chronic lung disease, and angina. He had his own albuterol inhaler, nitroglycerin tabs, and aspirin, but had not taken any because they were upstairs in the medicine chest.

Critical Thinking 2: Read the scenario. Determine which drug the patient should have, give at least one reason for the patient to have that drug, and list the things that must be reassessed after giving the drug.

Joel and Rick had been called for a woman having difficulty breathing. When they arrived, they found her seated in a chair with a very anxious look on her face. She was flushed in appearance with a raised rash on her face, neck, and arms. Her friends reported that they had been outside playing tennis when a ball went out of bounds into the brush. When the patient came from retrieving it, she complained of a stinging sensation on her leg. Soon after, her speech became thick, and she complained of being dizzy. An exam showed extensive wheezing in both lungs. The friends showed Rick the patient's medications, which included an autoinjector of epinephrine, a metered dose inhaler without a drug name on it, and an antismoking patch.

Critical Thinking 3: Read the scenario. Determine which drug the patient should have, give at least one reason for the patient to have that drug, and list the things that must be reassessed after giving the drug.

Sean and Todd went to the home of a middle-aged woman who complained of having difficulty breathing. When they arrived there, they found her holding her chest. She said she could not get enough air in because it felt like an elephant was seated on her chest. Her past medical history included asthma, diabetes, and angina. The physical exam showed an open airway and clear lungs, with vital signs of BP 134/80, pulse 96, and regular and nonlabored respirations of 18. She had not taken any of her medications, which included nitro tabs, an albuterol inhaler, and insulin.

Student Name _____ Date _____

Skill 22–1: Use of Metered Dose Inhaler

Purpose: To administer a dose of prescribed bronchodilator medication to the patient.

Standard Precautions:
- Gloves
- Goggles
- Mask

Equipment Needed:

1. Prescribed metered dose inhaler
2. Oxygen

Yes: ❑   Reteach: ❑   Return: ❑   Instructor initials: _____

Step One: Ensure scene safety, and apply appropriate personal protective equipment prior to assessing patient.

Yes: ❑   Reteach: ❑   Return: ❑   Instructor initials: _____

Step Two: Assess patient and apply oxygen, as appropriate.

Yes: ❑   Reteach: ❑   Return: ❑   Instructor initials: _____

Step Three: Confirm "rights."

Yes: ❑   Reteach: ❑   Return: ❑   Instructor initials: _____

Step Four: Shake inhaler.

Yes: ❑   Reteach: ❑   Return: ❑   Instructor initials: _____

Step Five: Remove mouthpiece cover.

Yes: ❑   Reteach: ❑   Return: ❑   Instructor initials: _____

Step Six: Ask patient to exhale, then to inhale slowly and deeply. Remove oxygen mask.

Yes: ❑   Reteach: ❑   Return: ❑   Instructor initials: _____

(continues)

Skill 22–1: Continued

Step Seven: Place inhaler to patient's mouth; at onset of inhalation, depress canister to release one puff of aerosolized medication.

Yes: ❏   Reteach: ❏   Return: ❏   Instructor initials: _____

Step Eight: Remove inhaler from patient's mouth, reapply oxygen, and instruct the patient to continue the inhalation and that he should hold his breath for several seconds.

Yes: ❏   Reteach: ❏   Return: ❏   Instructor initials: _____

Step Nine: Wait one minute, then repeat procedure.

Yes: ❏   Reteach: ❏   Return: ❏   Instructor initials: _____

Step Ten: Reevaluate patient.

Yes: ❏   Reteach: ❏   Return: ❏   Instructor initials: _____

Student Name _____ Date _____

Skill 22–2: Epinephrine Auto-injector Administration

Purpose: To assist the patient with administration of epinephrine by auto-injector in a case of anaphylaxis.

Standard Precautions:
- Hand washing
- Gloves

Equipment Needed:

1. Oxygen
2. Airway and ventilation equipment standing by
3. Prescribed epinephrine auto-injector

Yes: ❏ Reteach: ❏ Return: ❏ Instructor initials: _____

Step One: Ensure scene safety, and apply appropriate personal protective equipment prior to assessing patient.

Yes: ❏ Reteach: ❏ Return: ❏ Instructor initials: _____

Step Two: Assess patient and apply oxygen, as appropriate.

Yes: ❏ Reteach: ❏ Return: ❏ Instructor initials: _____

Step Three: Determine need for epinephrine, and confirm presence of auto-injector.

Yes: ❏ Reteach: ❏ Return: ❏ Instructor initials: _____

Step Four: Bare patient's lateral thigh.

Yes: ❏ Reteach: ❏ Return: ❏ Instructor initials: _____

Step Five: Follow instructions on auto-injector to remove safety mechanism.

Yes: ❏ Reteach: ❏ Return: ❏ Instructor initials: _____

Step Six: Press auto-injector firmly against the patient's lateral thigh, midway between knee and hip, allowing 10 seconds for medication administration.

Yes: ❏ Reteach: ❏ Return: ❏ Instructor initials: _____

(continues)

Skill 22–2: Continued

Step Seven: Remove the injector and properly dispose of it.

Yes: ❏   Reteach: ❏   Return: ❏   Instructor initials: _____

Step Eight: Initiate transport, if not already done, and reassess patient.

Yes: ❏   Reteach: ❏   Return: ❏   Instructor initials: _____

CHAPTER 23 SHORTNESS OF BREATH

Difficulty breathing can be caused by many different problems. Each of these problems may result from a different disease, even though they all cause dysfunction of the respiratory system.

Word Scramble: From the Key Terms found in Chapter 23 of the textbook, unscramble the following words.

1. hasmat   _____
2. oobcarmpsh   _____
3. eacclrks   _____
4. pruco   _____
5. scaysoni   _____
6. idisfonuf   _____
7. peadsny   _____
8. tttiiipegols   _____
9. corhnhi   _____
10. ezghwine   _____

Fill in the Blank: Complete each of the following statements.

1. When in distress, a patient will use _____ _____ of _____, located in the chest and neck to help with breathing.

2. _____ _____ _____ _____ describes the movement of oxygen and carbon dioxide between the lungs and the blood.

3. The process allowing the exchange of gas in the periphery is _____ _____.

4. _____ _____ _____ _____, or COPD, is a group of diseases characterized by airway obstruction and bronchospasm.

5. Back up of pressure from the left side of the heart causing fluids to leak into the alveoli describes _____ _____ _____.

6. Low levels of oxygen stimulate breathing in a patient on _____ _____.

7. A blockage in the pulmonary arterial circulation disrupting gas exchange is called a _____ _____.

8. Gas exchange is called _____, while movement of air in and out of the lungs is _____.

Sorting: List the characteristics found in children, adults, or both by placing each in the correct category.

very flexible trachea	floppy large epiglottis	15–30 breaths per minute
easily obstructed by slight swelling	tongue takes up most of mouth	wheezing
12–20 breaths per minute		

Pediatric   **Adult**   **Both**

Matching: Match word or words with its definition. Place the letter of the correct definition on the line in front of the term.

1. _____ croup
2. _____ epiglottitis
3. _____ pulmonary embolus
4. _____ CHF
5. _____ COPD
6. _____ asthma
7. _____ dyspnea

a. feeling it is difficult to breathe
b. hyperreactive airway disease
c. viral infection of kids causing barking cough
d. infection of tissues above the larynx
e. airways open, blood flow in lungs impaired
f. chronic disorder of airways
g. fluid-filled alveoli

Short Answer: For each of the diseases, list at least one risk factor.

1. Pulmonary embolus
2. COPD
3. Asthma
4. Croup
5. Epiglottitis

Completion: Complete the following drug card for an albuterol inhaler.

Generic name   albuterol
Trade name
Indication
Contraindication
Dose
Route

Labeling: Identify the following structures on the diagram.

Nose
Mouth
Pharynx
Larynx
Trachea
Right lung
Bronchus
Bronchiole
Alveoli

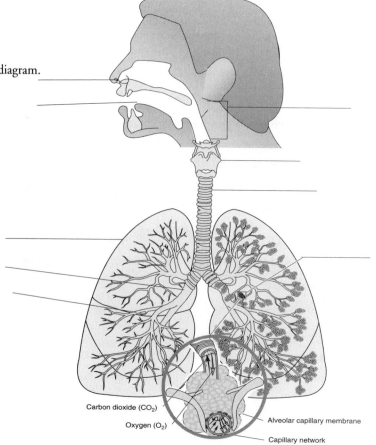

Carbon dioxide (CO_2)
Oxygen (O_2)
Alveolar capillary membrane
Capillary network

Short Answer: Answer the following from your readings.

1. Why does the body eventually switch to hypoxic drive?

2. Explain why the body doesn't switch to hypoxic drive in hypoperfusion.

Critical Thinking 1: Read the scenario and answer the questions at the end.

As the weather got colder, Diane and Jim found themselves answering more and more calls for difficulty breathing. This was the one they feared. Dispatch was for a 2-year-old experiencing difficulty in breathing. When they arrived, they found a calm but worried mother holding her 2-year-old daughter, Kara. Kara's wheezing could be heard without a stethoscope. She had a cold that had gotten worse over the course of last evening. Her mother had tried to manage it with prescribed medications and mist from the shower in the bathroom. Kara had continued to get worse, and so 911 was called.

While Jim asked Kara's mother questions, Diane applied oxygen and continued her assessment. Kara had a history of asthma and normally took ventolin syrup, and could be given a nebulizer treatment of ventolin by her mother as well. She was otherwise a healthy, happy little girl. When Kara's asthma was diagnosed, her family had given their kitten to the neighbors and Kara had not had an attack in over 6 months.

Diane and Jim moved Kara and her mother to the ambulance and strapped them in for safety. Diane began an ongoing assessment, and determined that Kara's respiratory rate had dropped from 32 breaths per minute to 12 per minute, and that the wheezing was very difficult to hear. Kara was also now difficult to awaken.

1. Why was Kara wheezing?

2. Why was Diane unable to hear wheezing when she continued her assessment?

3. What treatment must Diane begin now for Kara?

Critical Thinking 2: Read the scenario and answer the questions at the end.

Christina was a good EMT. When she heard her son Adam coughing during the night, she recognized the characteristic bark of croup. She also knew that she would need help. Adam had a cold for several days and was slightly feverish before he went to bed the previous evening. Now he was sounding like a seal and seemed to have difficult catching his breath.

Christina took him into the bathroom and turned on the shower while she called 911.

1. What produces the barking cough?

2. Should the responding EMTs examine inside Adam's mouth? Why or why not?

Critical Thinking 3: Read the scenario and answer the questions at the end.

Mr. Williamson called for EMS fairly often. He had a history of COPD and often found that he couldn't breathe well, even when taking his medication as prescribed. This time was far worse, however. By the time the EMTs had arrived, Mr. Williamson could hardly breathe at all!

While Jason began an initial assessment, Beth attempted to obtain a history. Mr. Williamson found it difficult to answer questions. Beth did discover that he had been exposed to some irritating vapors from a construction site nearby. Although it was quite cold out that day, the previous evening had been rather warm, and Mr. Williamson had kept his window open.

1. Should the EMTs administer oxygen to Mr. Williamson? Why or why not?

2. How should the EMTs prepare Mr. Williamson for transport?

CHAPTER 24 CHEST PAIN

EMT-Bs are frequently called to the scene of a patient experiencing chest pain. The accurate assessment and quick management of a patient with chest pain is the key to patient survival.

Definitions: Read each definition. Write the correct word or phrase on the line.

1. Pain produced by injured or dying heart muscle _____

2. Deposits of fat on the walls of arteries _____

3. Bulging veins of the neck (abbr) _____

4. Elevated BP _____

5. A blood clot _____

6. Arteries that provide blood to the heart muscle _____

7. Shock produced when the heart fails as a pump _____

8. The heart muscle _____

9. Blockage _____

10. Abnormally fast heart rate _____

11. Excessive perspiration due to stress or pain _____

12. Abdominal area just below the sternum _____

13. Abnormally slow heart rate _____

14. Circulation of oxygen and nutrients to cells _____

Identification: List eleven risk factors for cardiovascular disease. Place the risk factors in the correct column as modifiable or nonmodifiable.

Modifiable risk factors   **Nonmodifiable risk factors**

_____   _____

_____   _____

_____   _____

_____   _____

_____   _____

_____   _____

_____   _____

Labeling: Label the systemic and pulmonary circulations on the diagram below.

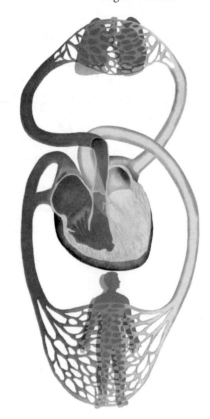

Identification: Read the common description given and write on the line the sign or symptom described.

1. Vise-like   _____

2. Toothache   _____

3. Heartburn   _____

4. Not enough oxygen   _____

5. No energy   _____

6. Cannot catch breath   _____

7. Dizzy   _____

8. Pressure   _____

9. Numbness/heaviness   _____

10. Indigestion   _____

True or False: Read each statement and decide if it is TRUE or FALSE. Place T or F on line before each statement.

1. _____ In assessing a patient with chest pain, it is not important to know what the patient was doing.

2. _____ Loss of consciousness is associated with cardiac problems.

3. _____ Neck and jaw pain are associated with cardiac chest pain.

4. _____ An older patient without a cardiac history is not likely having an MI.

5. _____ Cardiac pain always radiates to the left shoulder.

6. _____ Positional chest pain is highly indicative of a cardiac event.

7. _____ The therapeutic goal for a patient with chest pain is to reduce the pain by 50%.

8. _____ The EMT-B must ask about over-the-counter medications taken for pain.

9. _____ It is relatively uncommon for a young person to have a heart attack.

10. _____ Illicit drugs may lead to heart attacks in young adults.

Ordering: Place the following actions in the order in which they should be performed for a physical assessment of a patient complaining of chest pain. Put a numeral 1 before the first action, a 2 before the next, and so on.

_____ complete a focused physical exam

_____ assess the airway

_____ obtain baseline vital signs

_____ get a SAMPLE history

_____ survey the scene for safety

_____ check circulation

_____ note general impression

_____ assess breathing adequacy

Short Answer: Answer the following questions from your reading.

1. Why is it important for the EMT to provide early cardiac care?

2. Where does the heart muscle obtain its oxygen and nutrients?

3. Is it important for the EMT to be able to distinguish the diagnosis of angina from acute myocardial infarction?

Critical Thinking: Read the following scenario and answer the questions that follow.

Ambulance One responded to a call for a man with chest pressure. Mr. Stevens, 62 years old, had his wife call 911 after experiencing 2 hours of discomfort.

1. What are the components of the focused history and physical exam that should be performed on Mr. Stevens?

Mr. Stevens had a prescription for nitroglycerine. The EMTs assisted him in taking the medication.

2. What assessments must be made after Mr. Stevens takes the medication?

Five minutes after taking his nitroglycerine, Mr. Stevens complained of feeling dizzy. His blood pressure was 80/40.

3. How should the EMTs manage Mr. Stevens now?

CHAPTER 25 CARDIAC ARREST

In the not too distant past, cardiac arrest was a death sentence. However, advances in medicine and technology have made out-of-hospital arrest reversal more likely. EMTs, carrying special devices called automatic external defibrillators, are able to provide definitive care to the cardiac arrest victim.

Definitions: Write the definition of each word or phrase in the space provided.

1. defibrillation
2. dysrythmia
3. electrocardiogram
4. automaticity
5. rhythm
6. sudden cardiac death
7. chain of survival
8. public access defibrillation
9. artificial pacemaker
10. all clear command

Labeling: Label the sinoatrial node, the atrioventricular node, the Bundle of His, right and left bundle branches, the AV bundle, and the Purkinje fibers in the figure below.

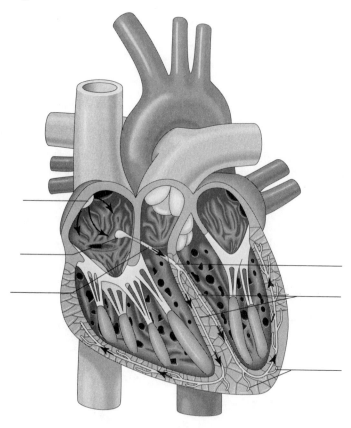

Identification: Identify each of the cardiac rhythms in Figures A, B, C, and D. Write the correct interpretation on the line.

A.

B.

C.

D.

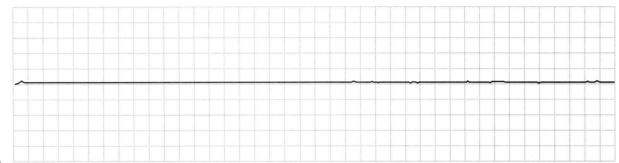

A.

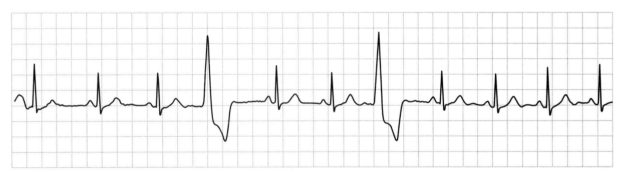

B.

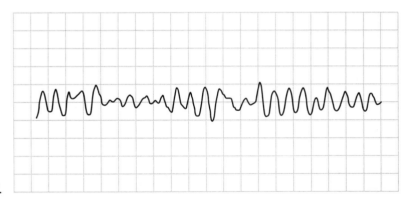

C.

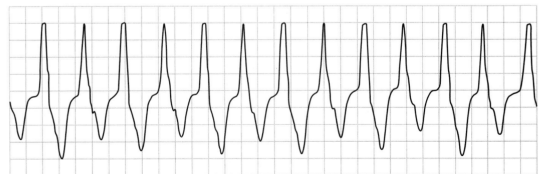

D.

Ordering: Place the following assessment into the correct order. Place a numeral 1 before the first thing to be done, 2 before the next, and so on.

_____ Open airway

_____ BSI/scene safety

_____ Check for carotid pulse

_____ Observe for chest rise

_____ Check responsiveness

Ordering: Place the following management techniques into the correct order. Place a numeral 1 before the first thing to be done, 2 before the next, and so on.

_____ Turn on AED and stop touching the patient

_____ Reanalyze/reassess

_____ Analyze rhythm

_____ Assess patient

_____ Apply patches/cable

_____ Clear patient for shock

_____ Press "shock" button

Identification: Read each of the following phrases. Decide if it is an indication for use of an AED, or a contraindication. Write the correct word on the line in front.

1. _____ Complaining of chest pain

2. _____ Thrashing

3. _____ Pulseless

4. _____ Airway blocked

5. _____ No carotid pulse

6. _____ No radial pulse while crying

7. _____ P on AVPU

8. _____ 5 years old

9. _____ mortal injuries

10. _____ pulseless, apneic, weighing 75 lbs

True or False: Read each sentence regarding safety and determine if it is TRUE or FALSE. Write T or F on the line before each statement.

1. _____ Using paddles for defibrillation gives the EMT better control of the procedure.

2. _____ Chest compressions can mimic ventricular fibrillation.

3. _____ Defibrillation should take place in a moving ambulance.

4. _____ "All clear" means that persons may touch the patient again.

5. _____ Do not defibrillate a patient who is in a puddle of water.

6. _____ It is acceptable for an EMT to override the suggestions of the AED.

7. _____ Be sure no one is touching the stretcher carriage during defibrillation.

8. _____ The operator of the AED is responsible for crew, bystander, and patient safety.

9. _____ Perform a head-to-toe sweep before discharging the AED.

10. _____ Move the AED pads away from an implanted pacemaker.

11. _____ Move a patient off a metal fire escape before defibrillating.

12. _____ Defib pads are effective when partially in contact with skin.

Short Answer: Answer the following questions from your reading.

1. Engineers can build smaller and more effective devices including AEDs. Why has no one designed a small AED for infants?

2. Why would the EMT still have patients to care for after someone is declared dead?

Critical Thinking 1: Read the following scenario and answer the questions that follow.

MaryLou and Chris arrived at the home of Mr. Roberts, a 50-year-old man who had collapsed in his front yard. His wife and daughter were performing CPR.

1. What should MaryLou and Chris do first?

2. Describe the necessary care for Mr. Roberts.

After the fourth shock, the AED read NO SHOCK ADVISED.

3. What should the EMTs do now?

Following ALS interventions by paramedics, Mr. Roberts is declared dead.

4. What care is necessary now?

Critical Thinking 2: Read the following scenario and answer the questions that follow.

The EMT supervisor arrived at the scene of a "cardiac problem." Bev and Joe were caring for a 62-year-old female, who was complaining of severe chest pain. They had placed her in a comfortable position, applied oxygen, and were in the process of applying the AED patches.

1. Do you agree with the care that was being provided?

2. If you were the EMT supervisor, how would you have handled this situation?

Student Name _____ Date _____

Skill 25–1: Operation of an Automated External Defibrillator

Purpose: To perform an external defibrillation, when indicated, to a patient in cardiac arrest.

Standard Precautions:
- Hand washing
- Gloves

Equipment Needed:

1. Automated external defibrillator

Yes: ❑   Reteach: ❑   Return: ❑   Instructor initials: _____

Step One: Confirm that the patient is in cardiac arrest.

Yes: ❑   Reteach: ❑   Return: ❑   Instructor initials: _____

Step Two: Apply the electrode pads to the anterior chest wall; one to the apex of the heart, and the other to the left sternal border below the clavicle.

Yes: ❑   Reteach: ❑   Return: ❑   Instructor initials: _____

Step Three: Turn the power on the AED while calling for "all clear." Ensure that no one is touching the patient.

Yes: ❑   Reteach: ❑   Return: ❑   Instructor initials: _____

Step Four: Press the analyze button and press the "shock" button, as advised. Again, the EMT must ensure that no one is touching the patient.

Yes: ❑   Reteach: ❑   Return: ❑   Instructor initials: _____

Step Five: After the series of shocks have been performed, check for the presence or absence of a pulse. If the pulse is absent, CPR must be continued for another minute.

Yes: ❑   Reteach: ❑   Return: ❑   Instructor initials: _____

Step Six: If the patient's pulse returns, check for breathing. If the patient's pulse does not return, then another round of shocks may be appropriate.

Yes: ❑   Reteach: ❑   Return: ❑   Instructor initials: _____

Chapter 26 Altered Mental Status

A patient may act confused, disoriented, or may "just not be acting right." The behavior may be due to illness, injury, or disease, and is called altered mental status. Several potentially dangerous medical conditions can create this, and the EMT must understand them and their management.

Matching: Match the word or words with its definition. Place the letter of the correct definition on the line in front of the term.

1. _____ aura		a.	one continuous seizure
2. _____ AEIOUTIPS		b.	old term for generalized seizure
3. _____ altered mental state		c.	diabetes occurring in pregnancy
4. _____ Alzheimer's disease		d.	old term for partial seizure
5. _____ anticonvulsant		e.	disease in which pancreas fails
6. _____ diabetes mellitus		f.	blood sugar control through eating habits
7. _____ diabetic coma		g.	drug to control seizures
8. _____ diet-controlled diabetes		h.	a progressive deterioration of brain function
9. _____ gestational diabetes		i.	drug that stimulates insulin production
10. _____ grand mal seizure		j.	unconscious patient with high blood sugar
11. _____ insulin shock		k.	a change in behavior
12. _____ amnesia		l.	a way to remember the causes of AMS
13. _____ status epilepticus		m.	failure to remember what happened
14. _____ petit mal seizure		n.	warning sign at the onset of a seizure
15. _____ oral hypoglycemic		o.	a low blood sugar

Correcting: Each of the following statements is false. Rewrite it to make it correct.

1. A person experiencing a change in behavior that may be due to illness or injury is having a psychiatric crisis.

2. A person who fails to remember what just happened is anaerobic.

3. Hypoglycemia is a lack of oxygen in the blood.

4. Diabetes mellitus occurs when the liver fails to produce sufficient insulin.

5. Excessive thirst is called polyuria.

6. The development of hyperglycemia is a sudden event, often occurring over minutes to an hour.

7. When the body cannot use sugar for energy, it uses ketoacids instead.

8. Kussmaul's respirations are slow and shallow.

9. Insulin shock results from excessive sugar in the blood.

10. A patient experiencing a low blood sugar will have warm, dry, flushed skin.

11. The cause of epilepsy is well-defined.

12. In a seizure affecting the whole brain, just a portion of the body is affected.

13. An origin is an odor or flash of light or sound that precedes certain seizures.

14. The post-ictal phase of a seizure occurs when the body stiffens.

15. Managing a seizing patient includes restraining the body.

Short Answer: Read each question and answer it from your reading.

1. Why will the brain "malfunction" when glucose is not available?

2. How can a person have diabetes mellitus and still produce insulin?

3. What is epilepsy? Name causes of seizures besides epilepsy.

4. Can someone have a seizure and still remain standing?

Critical Thinking 1: Read the following scenario and then answer the questions.

Bethany and Dean arrived on the scene of a bicycle accident to find a middle-aged man lying on the sidewalk next to his bike. Witnesses state that the man was "all over the place" just prior to taking a tumble. The witnesses could not figure out why the guy fell over; he didn't hit anything, and nothing was close to hit him.

Dean checked for responsiveness and took C-spine precautions to ensure that the neck and back stayed still. The man did not respond to Dean when he called to him. Bethany removed the bike helmet and completed an initial assessment. While looking for any signs of bleeding, she found a medic alert tag reading diabetes mellitus. No injuries were found during Bethany's exam. The man never responded to the touch or movements during the exam.

1. What do you think may have caused this incident?

2. How should the EMTs manage it?

3. Is the use of oral glucose indicated here? Why or why not?

Critical Thinking 2: Read the following scenario and then answer the questions.

The school nurse called EMS for a child actively seizing in the gymnasium. Upon arrival, Nora and Rich found a 10-year-old child lying on the mat beneath a climbing wall. The child was very still and snoring. The nurse related that the child had no significant medical history and was on no medications.

1. Name some likely causes of the child's current condition.

2. What safety precautions should the EMTs take to protect themselves and the child?

3. What measures must the EMTs take immediately during the initial assessment?

4. Is the use of oral glucose indicated here? Why or why not?

5. Is the use of oxygen indicated here? Why or why not?

Review glucose administration in Chapter 22.

CHAPTER 27 ABNORMAL BEHAVIOR

Mental illness is any disorder that affects the mind and is exhibited in a person's behavior. EMTs are less interested in the specific diagnoses of mental illness than in the behaviors that would generate an EMS call.

Matching: Match word or words with its definition. Place the letter of the correct definition on the line in front of the term.

1. _____ anxiety disorder
2. _____ dementia
3. _____ hallucination
4. _____ addiction
5. _____ withdrawal symptoms
6. _____ suicide
7. _____ mental illness
8. _____ dependency
9. _____ excited delirium
10. _____ delirium

a. sudden, erratic behavioral change
b. hyperactive irrational behavior
c. psychological need for a drug
d. unreal sensations or perceptions
e. nonphysical disorder that impairs brain function
f. voluntary taking of own life
g. gradual loss of ability to think
h. side effects of stopping some drugs
i. abnormal response to stress
j. physical need for a drug

Identification: Read each description and write the type of hallucination on the line.

1. _____ Sense of spiders walking on the skin
2. _____ God said to steal an item
3. _____ A mirage
4. _____ Sense of people talking about your clothes
5. _____ Perception that a clock is chiming
6. _____ Sense that Mom said to damage the car
7. _____ Sense that someone is touching your arm
8. _____ Sense that a dog is sitting there

Identification: Read each definition and write the correct name of the restraint device or action on the line.

1. _____ Holding or tying the arms and legs
2. _____ Heavy-duty, commercial wrist and ankle devices
3. _____ Totally encapsulating a patient
4. _____ Layering linens around a patient
5. _____ Planned, orderly method of subduing someone
6. _____ Suffocation resulting from an inability to breathe
7. _____ Minimum effort needed to confine a person
8. _____ Demonstration of determination
9. _____ Confined in order to protect the patient from harming himself

Sorting: Read each behavior listed and decide if the behavior is a behavioral emergency. Place a check mark in front of each instance that is a behavioral emergency. For each that is a behavioral emergency, describe how the EMT should handle the situation.

1. _____ A young mother is crying after the death of her infant.

2. _____ A teenager is threatening to shoot himself after getting a bad grade.

3. _____ A young man is crying loudly after he dropped his soda.

4. _____ A middle-aged woman is upset that she is having breathing difficulties.

5. _____ An elderly man is afraid that he will die if he enters a hospital.

6. _____ A young man threatens to kill all people who wear uniforms.

7. _____ A middle-aged man expresses anger that his wife just died.

8. _____ A newly arrived immigrant cannot follow a person's directions.

9. _____ A young man is upset after the saw he was using sliced his hand.

10. _____ A teenaged girl states she is going to stab all the snakes in the room.

True or False: Read each statement and decide if it is TRUE or FALSE. Place T or F on the line before each statement.

1. _____ You should only enter an unsafe scene during daylight hours.

2. _____ Always wear gloves when touching an object on a crime scene.

3. _____ Continually alert the dispatcher to what you are doing when approaching a potentially violent person.

4. _____ When walking with other EMTs, proceed side by side.

5. _____ An EMT can detect anger by the patient's posture.

6. _____ Rapid eye movements may indicate panic.

7. _____ The EMT should have an escape plan ready at all times.

8. _____ When gathering a history, the EMT should stand very close to the patient.

9. _____ Only one EMT should question the patient.

10. _____ The EMT should always speak louder than the patient.

Short Answer: Read each question and answer it from your reading.

1. Why is an adult patient experiencing a behavioral crisis not permitted to refuse restraints?

2. What is the minimum number of people required for a takedown? Why?

3. Once the patient is placed in the ambulance, where should the EMT sit to provide care? What tasks can be completed from this vantage point?

4. How often should pulses, movement, and sensation be checked in a restrained patient?

Critical Thinking 1: Read the scenario and then answer the questions that follow.

Geoff and Sandy responded to a call at Corner Ice Cream for a man acting strangely. It was not difficult to locate the man, as a large crowd of people had gathered in the parking lot. When they arrived, the man seemed to be mumbling words and striking out at thin air. Several of the onlookers were laughing and jeering at him, calling him an old drunk. Sandy requested a police unit to the scene and when it had arrived, Sandy and the officer carefully approached the patient. Geoff and the second officer watched the group of onlookers. The man was unable to answer questions; he just kept mumbling words. Neither Sandy nor the officer were able to detect any odor of an alcoholic beverage on him. Just when the man struck out at thin air, Sandy spied a medic alert tag detailing a history of diabetes.

1. Is this a behavioral emergency?

2. Is it likely that the cause of this situation is organic?

3. How should Geoff and Sandy proceed in the care of this man?

Critical Thinking 2: Read the scenario and then answer the questions that follow.

Security at the arena called for EMS to evaluate a man whose behavior seemed bizarre. Janie and Ralph responded, taking care to evaluate scene safety. The man was seated on the floor outside the men's lavatory. Every few minutes he would scream out that he "hated them and would jump and take them all with him."

1. Is there a behavioral emergency here?

2. How should Janie and Ralph approach this patient?

Janie spoke first to the patient. He told her that the voices kept telling him to do things, and he hated them. The voices, he said, told him that Janie was there to hurt him.

3. How should Janie react to the idea that she was trying to hurt the patient?

4. What should she say next?

5. Should Ralph speak with the patient? Why or why not?

The man agreed to go to the hospital. The security guard accompanied Janie in the back of the ambulance.

CHAPTER 28 ENVIRONMENTAL EMERGENCIES

In addition to exposure to the elements, water, and altitude, the EMT must be familiar with other emergencies, such as lightning strikes and bites, created by outdoor activities.

Matching: Match each of the following conditions with its description. Place the letter of the correct description on the line.

1. _____ chilblains
2. _____ trench foot
3. _____ frostnip
4. _____ frostbite
5. _____ hypothermia
6. _____ heat cramps
7. _____ heat exhaustion
8. _____ heat stroke
9. _____ bends
10. _____ air embolism
11. _____ HACE
12. _____ HAPE
13. _____ nitrogen narcosis
14. _____ near-drowning
15. _____ pulmonary over-pressurization syndrome

a. skin freezing

b. life-threatening heat illness

c. joint pain occurring after a rapid ascent

d. swelling of the brain from hypoxia at high altitudes

e. a reversible effect of breathing nitrogen

f. causes rupture of the alveoli

g. submersion not resulting in death within 24 hours

h. core body temperature below 95° F

i. inflamed area due to chronic cool and dampness

j. cough and dyspnea associated with high altitudes

k. painful muscle spasms from loss of fluids

l. tissue injury from chronic wet conditions

m. mild, generalized heat sickness with dehydration

n. air in a vessel resulting in a blockage of blood flow

o. local skin injury from freezing weather

Sorting: Read each action, and then place each in the category describing the specific type of heat loss.

Removing your sweater in a cool room

Sitting on cold rocks

Breathing

Sitting in front of a fan

Turning on the air conditioner in the house

Entering a meat cooler

Sweating

Swimming in a cold lake

Standing in the wind

Lying on a waterbed heated to 70° F

Radiation   **Convection**   **Conduction**   **Evaporation**

Identification: Place an X in front of those conditions that place persons at greater risk for hypothermia.

1. _____ diabetes mellitus
2. _____ adolescence
3. _____ heart disease
4. _____ multiple medications
5. _____ isolated broken wrist
6. _____ generalized infection
7. _____ burns

8. _____ sprained ankle
9. _____ thyroid condition
10. _____ head injury
11. _____ shock
12. _____ infected tooth
13. _____ spinal cord injury

Treatments: For each of the following conditions, list the management.

Local cold injuries

Hypothermia

Heat cramps

Heat exhaustion

Heat stroke

Snake bites

Sorting: Place an X in front of those signs or symptoms seen in hypothermia.

1. _____ poor coordination
2. _____ flushing
3. _____ nausea
4. _____ slurred speech
5. _____ poor judgment
6. _____ slow pulse

7. _____ pale skin
8. _____ stomach cramps
9. _____ mood changes
10. _____ decreased sensation
11. _____ muscle cramps
12. _____ itching

Identification: Which of these are active measures of rewarming, and which are passive? Place the answer on the line in front of each.

1. _____ heat packs to groin
2. _____ blankets
3. _____ hot water bottles to arms
4. _____ shelter from wind

5. _____ removing wet clothing
6. _____ hot drinks
7. _____ heating pads
8. _____ hat on head

Ordering: Place the following methods for water rescue in order of priority, putting a numeral 1 before the first step, 2 before the next, and so on.

_____ row   _____ go

_____ reach   _____ throw

Listing: List the types of incidents (injuries) that occur at each phase of diving.

Descent

Ascent

Fill in the Blank: Complete the following paragraph regarding lightning strikes.

Lightning strikes are divided into _____ and _____ injuries. With lesser injuries, the common symptoms include _____, _____, and short-term memory difficulties. A large percentage of people suffer ruptured _____. They may also suffer _____ trauma. The EMT should _____ the patient to prevent any further injuries.

   In other people, the electricity produces a shock that stops _____ electrical activity and a full arrest occurs. Even if the heart resumes function, the _____ may continue to malfunction, preventing _____ effort and resulting in hypoxia.

   The first priority in the management of a victim of a lightning strike is _____ _____.

Short Answer: Answer the following questions from your reading.

1. Name two major ways in which the body loses heat.

2. Describe how the body generates heat.

3. Describe two ways in which the body conserves heat.

4. Give two reasons why the elderly and very young cannot protect themselves against the extremes of heat and cold.

5. Explain how afterdrop occurs.

6. Name the complications of near-drowning.

7. How are diving emergencies related to drowning emergencies?

8. Why is oxygen indicated for managing mountain sickness?

Critical Thinking 1: Read the following scenario and answer the questions that follow.

Jessie and Anne responded to a call at a construction site for a man who had fallen off a scaffold. Upon their arrival, they found one man lying on wet ground and not moving, and three more confused and dazed. The foreman told them it was the most incredible scene he had ever witnessed. The four men were about 8 feet up when a freak storm hit. The rain was blinding, and the thunder resonated through the site. When it was over, Jay, his best employee, lay on the ground, and Jimmy, Ron, and Eric were acting strange.

1. What is the likely cause of this situation?

2. What is their first priority with this call?

3. Who should the EMTs care for first?

4. What other injuries must the EMTs be concerned with?

Critical Thinking 2: Read the following scenario and answer the questions that follow.

Debra and Brandon were sent to the home of Mrs. Miller, an 80-year-old woman living alone. The mailman had reported that Mrs. Miller was "not herself" today.

As they approached the home, a single-family bungalow in a quiet section of town, they remarked on the sudden cold snap. It was only September, but it seemed more like December in the Northeast. The mailman was waiting outside the home for the EMTs, and he commented on how well Mrs. Miller had seemed yesterday. Brandon noticed that all first-floor windows in the house were open.

Mrs. Miller was sitting on her couch. Her speech was slurred and she seemed unable to move easily. Her arms and torso were cold to the touch.

1. What do the EMTs know about this event?

2. How should they proceed?

Critical Thinking 3: Read the following scenario and answer the questions that follow.

It was late October, and George realized he was late in bringing wood in for the stove. While stacking wood next to the wood-pile, he felt a pinch on his leg. Not being a man to complain, he continued working until the swelling became too bad. Now, he had severe stomach pain and a very weak feeling.

1. What likely happened to George?

2. How should the EMTs manage care for him?

3. Should George be seen at a hospital?

CHAPTER 29 POISONING AND ALLERGIC REACTIONS

Exposure to substances with deadly ingredients can cause predictable or unpredictable reactions. It is important for the EMT to be familiar with the concepts of poisonings and allergic reactions, and understand their priorities and management.

Matching: Match the word or words with its definition. Place the letter of the correct definition on the line in front of each.

1. ___ allergen
2. ___ anaphylaxis
3. ___ overdose
4. ___ stridor
5. ___ urticaria
6. ___ reaction
7. ___ poison control
8. ___ charcoal
9. ___ 20 minutes
10. ___ 30 minutes

a. hives
b. prevents the absorption of some substances
c. amount of time that eyes should be flushed
d. causes activation of immune system
e. time when an allergic reaction normally starts
f. serious allergic reaction that leads to shock
g. often indicative of vocal chord swelling
h. response to allergen
i. resource regarding various substances
j. often deliberate overexposure to drug

Definitions: Write the definition for each of the following in the space provided.

1. allergic reaction

2. epinephrine

3. ingestion

4. inhalation

5. injected

6. absorbed

7. poisoning

Identification: Identify each of the following as caused by injected, inhaled, absorbed, or ingested poisons.

1. Spider bite _____

2. Bee sting _____

3. Drain cleaner _____

4. Car exhaust _____

5. Chlorine gas _____

6. Poison ivy _____

7. Chemical fire extinguisher _____

8. Mace/pepper spray _____

9. Alcohol _____

10. Marijuana _____

True or False: Read each statement and decide if it is TRUE or FALSE. Place T or F on the line before each statement.

1. ____ Activated charcoal should be given only within one to two hours of ingesting a substance.

2. ____ Activated charcoal should be used only with patients who ingested caustic substances.

3. ____ Patients who are unconscious should be given activated charcoal.

4. ____ Activated charcoal is given in doses of 10 to 20 g for an adult.

5. ____ Adrenalin is another term for epinephrine.

6. ____ An EpiPen gives a dose of 0.3 to 0.5 mg.

7. ____ Stridor is an indication for use of activated charcoal.

Completion: Complete the following drug card for activated charcoal.

Generic name activated charcoal

Trade name

Indication

Contraindication

Dose

Route

Completion: Complete the following drug card for an epinephrine auto-injector.

Generic name Epinephrine

Trade name

Indication

Contraindication

Dose

Route

Short Answer: Read each question and answer it from your readings.

1. How do the assessment findings differ between a mild and a severe allergic reaction?

2. What are the signs that a patient with an allergic reaction is worsening?

Critical Thinking 1: Read the following scenario and answer the questions that follow.

An EMT performed CPR on a man's bare chest without using gloves. He later found that he had a pasty substance on his hands. The patient's wife stated that the patient uses nitroglycerin paste. The EMT is now feeling dizzy and lightheaded.

1. What is the route of exposure?

2. How should the EMTs manage it?

Critical Thinking 2: Read the following scenario and answer the questions that follow.

Meredith was mowing her lawn and disturbed a wasp's nest. She was stung repeatedly and stated, "I can't breathe." She had a high-pitched sound coming from her breathing.

1. What is the route of exposure?

2. How should the EMTs manage it?

Critical Thinking 3: Aimee was expecting company this evening and decided to give her apartment a good cleaning. To ensure it was clean, she mixed Clorox bleach with ammonia. She was then coughing and gagging.

1. What is the route of exposure?

2. How should the EMTs manage it?

CHAPTER 30 HEAD INJURIES

Approximately half of the trauma deaths in the United States are due to head injuries. Recognition of the signs and symptoms of a serious head injury is a necessary skill for an EMT. It is crucial that the EMT be familiar with the concepts of managing a patient with a head injury.

Matching: Match the word or words with the correct definition. Place the letter of the correct definition on the line in front of the term.

1. _____ basilar skull fracture
2. _____ Cushing's reflex
3. _____ Cushing's triad
4. _____ Glascow Coma Scale
5. _____ intracranial pressure
6. _____ mastoid process
7. _____ subdural hematoma
8. _____ epidural hematoma
9. _____ posttraumatic seizure
10. _____ hematoma

a. a way to quantify level of consciousness
b. bony prominence behind the ear
c. a collection of blood
d. blood between the brain and the dura mater
e. seizing after head trauma
f. pressure within the skull
g. break at the base of skull behind the face
h. hypertension/bradycardia after a head injury
i. blood between the skull and the dura mater
j. increased blood pressure, slow heart rate, and altered respiratory patterns after a serious head injury

Identification: Name the sign that is described by each of the following.

1. _____ Bruising over the mastoid process after a head injury
2. _____ CSF leaking from the ear
3. _____ Bruising around both eyes after a head injury
4. _____ CSF leaking from the nose
5. _____ Increased BP, decreased pulse, and irregular respirations after a head injury

True or False: Read each statement and decide if it is TRUE or FALSE. Place T or F on line before each statement.

1. _____ Examination of a fontanelle is an important assessment skill in both adults and children.
2. _____ The EMT should be able to differentiate a basilar skull fracture from an open one.
3. _____ In an open skull fracture, cover the exposed brain with a saline-soaked dressing.
4. _____ Stabilize an object that has penetrated the skull.
5. _____ The elderly are at increased risk of developing a subdural hematoma after minor trauma.
6. _____ If changes in level of consciousness occur more than 24 hours after the injury, the patient has suffered an epidural hematoma.
7. _____ Bleeding inside the skull can occur in the absence of trauma.
8. _____ The EMT should suspect spinal injury with head trauma.
9. _____ Persistent vomiting is associated with serious head injury.
10. _____ A patient can receive a total of zero (0) on the Glasgow Coma Scale.

Calculation: Calculate the Glascow Coma Score for each of the following.

1. When called to, patient opens eyes, mumbles sounds, and moves hand away when pinched

2. The patient watches what the EMTs are doing, asks questions about care, and extends arm when told the EMT will take a blood pressure

3. Patient's eyes are closed, makes no sounds, and extends arms and legs stiffly when pinched

4. The patient makes no movement or sounds

5. Patient looks at EMT when spoken to, doesn't know where he is, keeps asking about incident, and pushes the EMT's hand away when pinched

Sorting: Place an X in front of each intervention appropriate to a significantly head-injured patient.

_____ ventilate at up to 20 breaths per minute in the adult patient

_____ elevate the head of the stretcher or board

_____ stop CSF flow

_____ control bleeding

_____ determine exact diagnosis

_____ withhold oxygen

_____ provide rapid transport

_____ avoid helicopter transport due to pressure changes

_____ calculate GCS

Fill in the Blank: Complete the following.

The most important thing an EMT can do to improve the outcome of a head-injured patient is to adequately assess and manage the _____, _____, and _____ status. The brain needs adequate perfusion with well-_____ blood. After ensuring an adequate airway, assess the effectiveness of the patient's own _____. Next, turn attention to the _____ status.

For the patient who has suffered a significant injury, the EMT should then move on to a _____ _____ _____. For a high-priority patient, this will be done during transport. During both assessments completed up to this time, the _____ of _____, or patient responsiveness, will be observed. This can be quantified on the _____ _____ scale. A _____ or pattern that may be seen in repeated vital signs is an increased BP, decreased pulse rate, and changed respiratory pattern. This combination is called _____ _____.

As with all high priority patients, be sure the patient is receiving high-_____ _____. Ongoing assessments should be completed every 5 minutes.

Short Answer: Answer the following questions.

1. Why is hypotension so dangerous for a patient with a head injury?

2. What causes the fontanelles to bulge?

Critical Thinking 1: Read the following scenario and answer the questions that follow.

Janice and Brad were assigned to standby at the motorcross rally. They were enjoying the sport when the radio crackled. There was accident on the first hill. A 12-year-old named Billy was lying on the ground, not moving. Spectators reported that he had missed a jump and struck a tree head first. His helmet, which was nearby, was cracked.

1. Based on the report, what injuries should the EMTs suspect?

2. What interventions must be provided for Billy during the initial assessment?

3. What two methods should the EMTs use to document mental status?

4. List two methods the EMTs can use to reduce brain swelling.

Critical Thinking 2: Read the following scenario and answer the questions that follow.

Carolyn's mother was upset as she spoke to the EMTs. She and Carolyn were shopping at the mall when Carolyn suddenly collapsed, striking her head hard on the floor. She appeared to have had a seizure. Mall security reported that Carolyn was unresponsive when they first arrived, then awoke briefly and talked with them, complaining of a headache. Now she was unresponsive again.

1. What initial management must be provided for Carolyn?

2. List eight signs of increasing intracranial pressure.

3. What treatment do you expect will occur at the hospital?

CHAPTER 31 SPINE INJURIES

The immediate care provided to the patient with a spinal injury is critical to prevent further damage from occurring. An EMT is often the primary prehospital caregiver for patients who have sustained spine injuries. It is important that the EMT knows how to recognize that a spinal injury may exist, and how to properly care for such a patient.

Word Scramble: Unscramble the following words using the Key Terms found in Chapter 31 of the textbook.

1. Inability to move   ssaalypri   _____
2. Cannot move lower extremities   geapipaarl   _____
3. Abnormal sensation   reetasisaph   _____
4. Cannot move four extremities   idregquiplaa   _____
5. Caused by nerve interruption   spaimipr   _____

Identification: Complete the following anatomy review.

_____   Bones of the spinal column

_____   First seven bones of column compose the ___ spine

_____   Portion of the spine behind the chest

_____   Part of spine considered low back

_____   Coverings over cord and brain

Fill in the Blank: Fill in the blanks in the following.

The first clue the EMT has as to the possibility of a spinal injury is the _____ of _____. Knowing the stacked nature of the vertebrae will enable the EMT to imagine the injuries. In a motor vehicle collision, the most common injury type is _____ of the neck. Falls can result in _____ bones that intrude into the cord, or _____ fractures that actually crush the vertebrae. The phenomenon, known as _____ _____, can cause trauma along the spinal column, especially in the lumbar region. Firearms can lead to spinal injuries due to the uncertainty of the _____ of _____ of the bullet. Sports injuries may also cause spinal injury.

True or False: Read each sentence regarding spinal injuries and determine if it is TRUE or FALSE. Write T or F on the line.

1. _____ All spinal injuries will result in nerve deficit.
2. _____ The first clue to a spinal injury is the MOI.
3. _____ Suspicion of spinal injury should be much higher in the elderly.
4. _____ Patients with gunshot injuries to neck or torso should be treated as if they have a spinal cord injury.
5. _____ Alcohol use increases the sensations associated with spinal injury.
6. _____ The inability to move is called paresthesia.
7. _____ Neurogenic shock is characterized by a slow heart rate and warm skin.
8. _____ The first priority of care in a suspected spinal cord injury is to protect the cord.
9. _____ A cervical spine immobilization device is a definitive method of spinal protection.
10. _____ Rapid extrication is for all persons with suspected spinal cord injury.

166

Short Answer: Answer the following.

1. Explain how it is possible for a patient with a broken vertebra to walk around immediately after an incident.

2. A patient tells you that he has broken his tailbone. Is this possible? Why or why not? Would this result in a spinal cord deficit?

3. Why would a spinal injury in the neck cause greater management difficulties for the EMT than an identical injury located in the lumbar area?

4. Why does a patient with neurogenic shock present differently than one with hypovolemic shock?

5. How would the suspicion of a spinal cord injury alter airway management?

Critical Thinking: Read each of the scenarios and decide how to manage the patient's spine.

1. A 45-year-old man was involved in a low-speed, rear-end collision. He is complaining of neck and shoulder pain. He was wearing both a lap and shoulder harness, he had full movement and sensation of lower extremities, and there was minimal damage to either car.

2. An unrestrained female was involved in a head-on collision into a tree. There were no skid marks, a posted speed limit 40 mph, and she had difficulty breathing.

3. An 18-year-old male was walking around his damaged Jeep. Vehicle rolled twice on highway, ending up in a ditch. The driver couldn't remember if he was wearing a seat belt. He denies complaints.

Student Name _____ Date _____

Skill 31–1: Application of the Cervical Immobilization Device

Purpose: To aid the EMT in stabilization of cervical spine.

Standard Precautions:
- Hand washing
- Gloves

Equipment Needed:

1. Assortment of cervical immobilization devices (collars)

Yes: ❑   Reteach: ❑   Return: ❑   Instructor initials: _____

Step One: Move the patient's head into neutral alignment. If the patient complains of pain, or resistance is felt, then the patient's neck should be splinted in position.

Yes: ❑   Reteach: ❑   Return: ❑   Instructor initials: _____

Step Two: Assign a trained assistant to maintain continuous manual stabilization of the patient's head.

Yes: ❑   Reteach: ❑   Return: ❑   Instructor initials: _____

Step Three: Check for distal pulses, movement, and sensation.

Yes: ❑   Reteach: ❑   Return: ❑   Instructor initials: _____

Step Four: Measure the patient's neck for cervical collar, according to manufacturer recommendations.

Yes: ❑   Reteach: ❑   Return: ❑   Instructor initials: _____

Step Five: Slide the posterior portion of collar in the void behind the neck.

Yes: ❑   Reteach: ❑   Return: ❑   Instructor initials: _____

Step Six: Cupping the chin piece in one hand, slide the anterior portion of the collar up the chest until it captures the chin.

Yes: ❑   Reteach: ❑   Return: ❑   Instructor initials: _____

(continues)

Skill 31–1: Continued

Step Seven: With collar in place, securely fasten the Velcro.

Yes: ❑   Reteach: ❑   Return: ❑   Instructor initials: _____

Step Eight: Checking for a proper collar fit, mentally draw a line from the opening of the ear to the middle of the shoulder, and from the opening of the ear to the eyes. There should be a 90-degree angle imagined.

Yes: ❑   Reteach: ❑   Return: ❑   Instructor initials: _____

Step Nine: Recheck for distal pulses, sensation, and movement.

Yes: ❑   Reteach: ❑   Return: ❑   Instructor initials: _____

Step Ten: Continuous manual stabilization must be maintained, despite the presence of the cervical immobilization device.

Yes: ❑   Reteach: ❑   Return: ❑   Instructor initials: _____

Student Name _____ Date _____

Skill 31–2: Application of the Short Immobilization Device

Purpose: To further immobilize the injured patient's spine after the application of the cervical collar.

Standard Precautions:

- Hand washing
- Gloves

Equipment Needed:

1. Assortment of cervical spine immobilization devices
2. Short immobilization device

Yes: ❏   Reteach: ❏   Return: ❏   Instructor initials: _____

Step One: Apply a properly sized cervical spine immobilization device after manually stabilizing the spine, as well as checking distal pulses, movement, and sensation.

Yes: ❏   Reteach: ❏   Return: ❏   Instructor initials: _____

Step Two: While a trained assistant maintains continuous manual stabilization, the EMT places his arms along the anterior and posterior thorax. The patient may now be moved forward as a unit, keeping spine inline.

Yes: ❏   Reteach: ❏   Return: ❏   Instructor initials: _____

Step Three: The device is then positioned behind the patient cautiously; the patient is leaned back against the device.

Yes: ❏   Reteach: ❏   Return: ❏   Instructor initials: _____

Step Four: Next, the patient's torso, including the legs, is secured to the device.

Yes: ❏   Reteach: ❏   Return: ❏   Instructor initials: _____

Step Five: Finally, the patient's head is secured to the device. The EMT pads the void behind the head as needed.

Yes: ❏   Reteach: ❏   Return: ❏   Instructor initials: _____

Step Six: The EMT then reassesses distal pulses, movement, and sensory function of the patient before transferring the patient to the backboard.

Yes: ❏   Reteach: ❏   Return: ❏   Instructor initials: _____

Student Name _____   Date _____

Skill 31–3: Rapid Extrication

Purpose: To manually immobilize the spine of an unstable patient who may have a spinal injury as a result of a motor vehicle collision.

Standard Precautions:
- Hand washing
- Gloves
- Turnout gear

Equipment Needed:

1. Assortment of cervical spine immobilization devices
2. Long spine board

Yes: ❑   Reteach: ❑   Return: ❑   Instructor initials: _____

Step One: The EMT first checks distal pulses, movement, and sensation. Then the EMT moves the head to a neutral position, and has another EMT apply a properly sized cervical collar.

Yes: ❑   Reteach: ❑   Return: ❑   Instructor initials: _____

Step Two: With an EMT on each side of the patient, the patient is gently lifted a couple of inches, so that a longboard may be inserted under the patient's buttocks.

Yes: ❑   Reteach: ❑   Return: ❑   Instructor initials: _____

Step Three: One EMT grasps the patient under the arms, while another grasps the patient at the hips. Then, on command, the EMTs rotate the patient to side about 45 degrees. At this point, the EMTs may need to switch places if the car's B post becomes an obstruction.

Yes: ❑   Reteach: ❑   Return: ❑   Instructor initials: _____

Step Four: Once the patient is parallel to the backboard, the patient is lowered, as a stiff unit, to the longboard, while the EMTs maintain inline immobilization.

Yes: ❑   Reteach: ❑   Return: ❑   Instructor initials: _____

Step Five: Once the patient is on the longboard, first the body and then the head should be fastened securely. The EMT should recheck the patient's distal pulses, movement, and circulation.

Yes: ❑   Reteach: ❑   Return: ❑   Instructor initials: _____

Student Name _____ Date _____

Skill 31–4: Long Axis Drag

Purpose: To rapidly remove a patient, who is in immediate danger, from a motor vehicle, with a minimum of spinal manipulation.

Standard Precautions:
- Hand washing
- Gloves
- Turnout gear

Equipment Needed:

None

Yes: ❑   Reteach: ❑   Return: ❑   Instructor initials: _____

Step One: First, the EMT determines that the patient needs immediate extrication for some reason; for example, if the patient is in cardiac arrest.

Yes: ❑   Reteach: ❑   Return: ❑   Instructor initials: _____

Step Two: Opening the closest door and entering the passenger compartment, the EMT disentangles any extremities from pedals and other obstructions.

Yes: ❑   Reteach: ❑   Return: ❑   Instructor initials: _____

Step Three: Then the EMT reaches behind the patient's back and, reaching under both of the patient's arms, grabs the wrists.

Yes: ❑   Reteach: ❑   Return: ❑   Instructor initials: _____

Step Four: The EMT then rotates the patient, as a unit, and places the patient into a semi-inclined position.

Yes: ❑   Reteach: ❑   Return: ❑   Instructor initials: _____

Step Five: The EMT then drags the patient out of the motor vehicle with the patient's head resting on the EMT's forearms.

Yes: ❑   Reteach: ❑   Return: ❑   Instructor initials: _____

Step Six: By dropping to his knees, the EMT can lower the patient and crawl backward with the patient, while performing a long axis drag.

Yes: ❑   Reteach: ❑   Return: ❑   Instructor initials: _____

Student Name _____   Date _____

Skill 31–5: Modified Logroll of the Supine Patient

Purpose: To immobilize the spine of a supine patient who may have a spinal injury.

Standard Precautions:
• Hand washing
• Gloves

Equipment Needed:

1. Selection of cervical collars
2. Long spine board
3. Strapping system
4. Head immobilization system

Yes: ❑   Reteach: ❑   Return: ❑   Instructor initials: _____

Step One: An EMT checks distal pulses, movement, and sensation of all four extremities, while another EMT maintains manual stabilization.

Yes: ❑   Reteach: ❑   Return: ❑   Instructor initials: _____

Step Two: While one EMT holds manual stabilization, two more take positions at the patient's shoulders and pelvis, reaching across the patient and grasping the patient's shoulders and pelvis, respectively.

Yes: ❑   Reteach: ❑   Return: ❑   Instructor initials: _____

Step Three: On command, the three EMTs roll the patient on his side. The patient's arms should be at his side.

Yes: ❑   Reteach: ❑   Return: ❑   Instructor initials: _____

Step Four: One EMT pulls the longboard under the patient. The longboard should end at the back of the patient's knees. The bottom of the longboard is at the patient's knees.

Yes: ❑   Reteach: ❑   Return: ❑   Instructor initials: _____

Step Five: On command, the patient is rolled back onto the longboard, and the patient is pulled up to the center of the board, using a long axis drag.

Yes: ❑   Reteach: ❑   Return: ❑   Instructor initials: _____

Step Six: Once the patient is centered on the longboard, the EMT secures the patient to the longboard and reassesses distal pulses, movement, and sensation.

Yes: ❑   Reteach: ❑   Return: ❑   Instructor initials: _____

Student Name _____ Date _____

Skill 31–6: Four Person Lift

Purpose: To immobilize the spine of a supine patient who may have a spinal injury.

Standard Precautions:
- Hand washing
- Gloves

Equipment Needed:

1. Assortment of cervical collars
2. Long spine board
3. Strapping system
4. Head immobilization system

Yes: ❏   Reteach: ❏   Return: ❏   Instructor initials: _____

Step One: The first EMT kneels at the patient's head and immediately obtains manual stabilization. The second EMT checks the patient's distal pulses, movement, and sensation, and applies a cervical collar.

Yes: ❏   Reteach: ❏   Return: ❏   Instructor initials: _____

Step Two: The second EMT then straddles the patient and drops one knee to the ground. Placing his hands under the patient's arms, he grasps the shoulder girdle.

Yes: ❏   Reteach: ❏   Return: ❏   Instructor initials: _____

Step Three: A third EMT straddles the patient at the hips and drops his opposite knee to the ground. He then grasps the patient around the hips.

Yes: ❏   Reteach: ❏   Return: ❏   Instructor initials: _____

Step Four: On command, three EMTs gently and evenly lift the patient about 2 inches, while a fourth EMT slides the longboard under the patient.

Yes: ❏   Reteach: ❏   Return: ❏   Instructor initials: _____

Step Five: Once the patient is properly positioned, the EMTs proceed to immobilize the torso, and then the head of the patient. Then the EMT rechecks distal pulses, movement, and sensation.

Yes: ❏   Reteach: ❏   Return: ❏   Instructor initials: _____

Student Name _____   Date _____

Skill 31–7: Longboard Immobilization of the Standing Patient

Purpose: To immobilize the spine of a supine patient who may have a spinal injury.

Standard Precautions:
- Hand washing
- Gloves

Equipment Needed:

1. Assortment of cervical collars
2. Long spine board
3. Strapping system
4. Head immobilization system

Yes: ❑   Reteach: ❑   Return: ❑   Instructor initials: _____

Step One: The EMT approaches the patient from the front and takes immediate anterior head stabilization.

Yes: ❑   Reteach: ❑   Return: ❑   Instructor initials: _____

Step Two: Another EMT takes head stabilization from the rear, while the first EMT assesses distal pulses, movement, and sensation.

Yes: ❑   Reteach: ❑   Return: ❑   Instructor initials: _____

Step Three: An appropriately sized cervical collar is applied to the patient.

Yes: ❑   Reteach: ❑   Return: ❑   Instructor initials: _____

Step Four: Another EMT places the longboard upright behind the patient and between the arms of the EMT holding stabilization.

Yes: ❑   Reteach: ❑   Return: ❑   Instructor initials: _____

Step Five: One EMT then stands on either side of the patient, holds the board under the patient's arms, and stabilizes the bottom of the board with a foot.

Yes: ❑   Reteach: ❑   Return: ❑   Instructor initials: _____

Step Six: Slowly, the board and the patient are lowered to the ground, while the EMT at the head stabilizes the head and neck. The EMT then immobilizes and rechecks distal pulses, movement, and sensation.

Yes: ❑   Reteach: ❑   Return: ❑   Instructor initials: _____

Student Name _____   Date _____

Skill 31–8: Helmet Removal

Purpose: To immobilize the spine of a patient who is wearing a full-face helmet, and may have a spine injury.

Standard Precautions:
- Hand washing
- Gloves

Equipment Needed:

1. Backboard
2. Scissors
3. Assortment of cervical collars

Yes: ❏   Reteach: ❏   Return: ❏   Instructor initials: _____

Step One: The first EMT manually stabilizes the head in the helmet, while the second EMT assesses distal pulses, movement, and sensation. Any glasses should be removed at this time.

Yes: ❏   Reteach: ❏   Return: ❏   Instructor initials: _____

Step Two: The second EMT then cuts the chin strap, slides one hand under the head, stabilizing the head from below, and places his hand on the jaw, stabilizing the head from above.

Yes: ❏   Reteach: ❏   Return: ❏   Instructor initials: _____

Step Three: The first EMT then removes the helmet by spreading the helmet apart gently, while moving the helmet from the back of the head.

Yes: ❏   Reteach: ❏   Return: ❏   Instructor initials: _____

Step Four: Once the helmet is completely removed, the first EMT assumes manual stabilization of the head. It may be necessary to pad under the head.

Yes: ❏   Reteach: ❏   Return: ❏   Instructor initials: _____

Step Five: A cervical collar is then fitted to the patient.

Yes: ❏   Reteach: ❏   Return: ❏   Instructor initials: _____

Step Six: With the collar in place, and the head in a neutral position, the EMT rechecks distal pulses, movement, and sensation.

Yes: ❏   Reteach: ❏   Return: ❏   Instructor initials: _____

CHAPTER 32 CHEST AND ABDOMINAL TRAUMA

Over one-half of all serious trauma patients have chest or abdominal injuries. Prehospital care provided by EMTs has a positive impact on the survival of these patients.

Missing Letters: Complete the puzzle using the Key Terms found in Chapter 32 of the textbook.

<pre>
cardiac   C _ _ _ _ _ _ _ _
          H _ _ _ _ _ _ _ _
          E _ _ _ _ _ _ _ _ _
sucking   _ _ _ S _ wound
          T _ _ _ _ _ _ _
          and
_ _ _ _ _ _ _ _ A _
          _ B _ _ _ _ _
_ _ _ _ D _ _ _ _ _ motion
_ _ _ _ O _ _ _ _ contusion
subcutaneous _ M _ _ _ _ _ _ _
          _ _ _ I _ segment
          _ _ N _ _ _ _ _ _ _ _ M _ _ _ _ _ _ _
_ _ _ _ _ _ _ A _
_ _ _ _ _ _ _ L deviation
          T _ _ _ _ _
</pre>

Identification: For each of the following signs or symptoms, state whether it is evidence of a simple pneumothorax (**S**), a tension pneumothorax (**T**), or both (**B**).

1. _____ Subcutaneous emphysema

2. _____ Tachycardia

3. _____ Tachypnea

4. _____ Difficulty breathing

5. _____ Diminished breath sounds

6. _____ Jugular venous distension

7. _____ Loss of radial pulses

8. _____ Decreased lung compliance

9. _____ Hypotension

10. _____ Tracheal deviation

Labeling: Label the following organs on the diagram below: heart, lungs, trachea, diaphragm, stomach, liver, small intestines, and bladder.

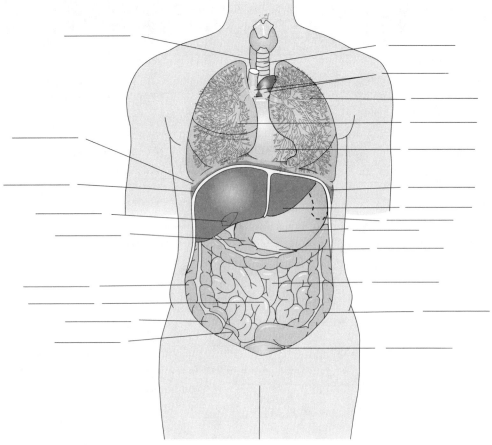

Completion: Complete each sentence.

1. The most common cause of serious chest injuries is _____ trauma.

2. Immediate results of penetrating trauma to the chest are impaired breathing and significant _____.

3. The most common signs and symptoms seen in patients with chest injuries are _____ and difficulty _____.

4. Use the mnemonic _____ to help look for injuries.

5. The sign best described as feeling like Rice Krispies is_____.

6. Management of chest injuries centers on ensuring adequate ventilation, _____, and _____.

7. Accumulation of blood in the pleural space is called _____.

8. The EMT should cover any open wounds to the chest with a(n) _____ _____.

9. Tape any occlusive dressings on _____ sides.

10. Transport the patient with a chest injury on the _____ side.

True or False: Read each statement and decide if it is TRUE or FALSE. Place a T or F on the line before each statement.

1. _____ A backup of blood from the heart can cause distended neck veins.

2. _____ A good method of splinting a fractured rib is to let the patient self-splint.

3. _____ Distended neck veins, petechiae, and altered mental status are signs of aortic rupture.

4. _____ Blunt trauma to the abdomen will cause eviscerations.

5. _____ Lower rib injuries may indicate underlying damage to bladder.

6. _____ Extrusion of the intestines outside the abdominal wall is called abdominal asphyxiation.

7. _____ The EMT must try to replace intestines that protrude through a wound.

8. _____ Moist, sterile dressings should be used to cover eviscerations.

9. _____ A major complication of pelvic fracture is hemorrhaging.

10. _____ Seat belts worn properly can leave contusions.

Short Answer: From your reading, answer the following questions.

1. Why is it unimportant for the EMT to diagnose the actual abdominal injury in the field?

2. Why is it important to cover exposed abdominal organs with moist, sterile dressings and a covering?

Critical Thinking: Read the following scenario and then answer the questions that follow.

Eve and James were dispatched to a local dance hall for "injuries following a fight, shots fired." The sheriff's patrol apprehended the shooter and secured the weapon. At the dance hall, the EMTs found a young man sitting in a chair, clutching his chest. He was screaming at the sheriff that they had better "put that guy away for life."

1. What do the EMTs know about their patient already?

The EMTs talked to the man while removing his shirt. He stated he was sitting in that chair when "this guy started screaming and waving a gun." Next thing he knew, he had been shot. James said he could visualize a small wound to the right side of the chest, approximately 10 inches below the patient's shoulder. There was a larger exit wound to the back in the same region.

2. What are the likely injuries?

3. How should the EMTs manage this patient?

4. How should he be transported?

During transport, he stated he could not breathe at all.

5. What should the EMTs do now?

CHAPTER 33 CUTS AND BLEEDING

Uncontrolled bleeding can lead to shock and even death. Fortunately, most bleeding is easily controlled using some very simple maneuvers.

Missing Letters: Complete each line by choosing the correct word or phrase from the terms found in Chapter 33 of the textbook.

C _ _ _ _ _ _ _ _

_ _ _ U _ _ _ _ _ _

_ _ _ _ T _ _ _

_ _ _ S _

_ _ _ A _ _ _ _

_ N _ _ _ _ _ _

_ _ _ _ _ _ D _ _ _ _ _ _

B _ _ _ _

_ _ _ L _ _ _ _

_ _ _ _ _ _ _ E

_ _ _ _ _ E _ _ _ _ _

_ _ _ _ D

_ _ _ _ _ _ _ I _ _ _

_ _ _ _ _ _ N _

_ _ G _ _ _ _ _ _

Identification: Read each of the following and then write on the line the name of the bandage or dressing described.

1. _____ A triangle folded into a band

2. _____ A strip of cloth that holds a dressing in place

3. _____ Sterile cotton weave cloth

4. _____ A 36" by 42", three-sided piece of cloth

5. _____ Any sterile, absorbent cloth

6. _____ A circumferential cloth holding a chest dressing

7. _____ An added layer that directly pushes on the wound

8. _____ A cylinder of cloth continually folding back onto itself

9. _____ An impenetrable covering

10. _____ A cotton dressing with two tails for tying

11. _____ Cloth laid back and forth across tape, then anchored

12. _____ A cylinder of cloth used for ease in application

13. _____ A cylinder of cloth applied around a limb

14. _____ A 9" by 36" multilayered cloth

15. _____ A constricting band

Definitions: Write the definition of each word in the space provided.

1. hemorrhage

2. inflammation

3. necrotic

4. coagulation

5. ecchymosis

6. embolism

7. fasciotomy

True or False: Read each statement and decide if it is TRUE or FALSE. Place T or F on the line before each statement.

1. _____ Bleeding can lead to shock.

2. _____ The first step in controlling bleeding is elevation.

3. _____ A tourniquet is useful for controlling capillary bleeding.

4. _____ The pressure point is located within the wound itself.

5. _____ To adequately compress blood vessels, apply an occlusive dressing.

6. _____ Elevation decreases pressure in the vessels serving the wound area.

7. _____ BSI is necessary when caring for a wound.

8. _____ If blood seeps through the first dressing, take it off and apply a new one.

Sorting: Place each descriptor of bleeding into the correct category.

constant   pulsing

watery   pouring out of wound

seeping   oozing

spurting   bright red

deep red   rivulets

Arterial bleeding   **Venous bleeding**   **Capillary bleeding**

Calculation: Using the rule of nines or the palmer method, calculate the percentage of burn.

1. The entire right leg of an adult

2. The front of both arms, front of the chest, and front of the abdomen of an adult

3. Front and back of both legs and the genitalia of a one-year-old child

4. The bottom of the foot of an adult

5. Back of the chest and lower back of an adult

6. A child's palm

7. Entire head of a child

8. The entire left leg, abdomen, and front of left arm of an adult

9. A 2" by 3" section on the front of an adult's abdomen

10. Front of the neck, face, and half of the top of the head on an adult

Identification: Write the correct classification of burn on the line.

1. _____ Reddened

2. _____ Little damage to living tissue

3. _____ Charred

4. _____ Swollen

5. _____ Destruction of nerve endings

6. _____ Painless

7. _____ Leathery

8. _____ Loss of muscle and fat

9. _____ Blistered

10. _____ Flat but painful

Short Answer: Answer each of the following questions.

1. A patient receives a partial thickness burn from hot steam used to sterilize equipment. Why is he at risk for infection?

2. Why is it important to concentrate on finding all injuries, instead of just locating the exit and entrance wounds from a gunshot?

3. An EMT is taught to leave an impaled object in place. What can happen if it is removed?

4. Regarding an impaled object, why is the cheek treated differently?

Critical Thinking 1: Read this scenario and answer the questions at the end.

Kim and Christina were dispatched to the local industrial park for a worker injured and bleeding. Upon their arrival, they found Mark, a 24-year-old laborer, sitting on a pallet holding onto his neck. The front of his shirt was dark red. The local police were also on scene. Mark's foreman had been opening boxes, when he hit a metal tie. This caused the razor to slip and he hit Mark with it. Kim and Christina took BSI and began their initial assessment.

1. What are the two major concerns for Mark at this point?

2. What treatments must the EMTs provide for Mark during the initial assessment?

3. Once they provide those treatments, why is Mark at great risk for hypoxia?

Critical Thinking 2: Read this scenario and answer the questions at the end.

Genna and Andy were staged around the corner from a domestic fight. The dispatch information was that one adult had been stabbed in the chest with an ice pick. The EMTs discussed the likely injuries to result from such an incident. Genna mentioned that they needed to carefully assess for air moving in and out of the chest wound.

1. What type of wound has occurred if air is moving in and out of the chest through the wound?

2. What problems are present for the patient with this type of injury?

3. What treatments must Genna and Andy provide for the patient if this type of injury is present?

Chapter 34 Bony Injuries

Most bone injuries are not life-threatening. Careful attention by the EMT to the assessment and management of bone injuries can reduce suffering, prevent further injury, and ultimately assist the patient to a return to health.

Identification: Refer to Chapter 5 to complete the following exercise. List the important bones in each region of the body.

1. Upper and lower arm

2. Wrist and hand

3. Upper and lower leg

4. Ankle and foot

5. Trunk

Definitions: Write the definition of each of the following words or terms.

1. closed fracture   _____

2. dislocation   _____

3. dorsiflexion   _____

4. footdrop   _____

5. locked   _____

6. motor nerves   _____

7. open fracture   _____

8. osteoporosis   _____

9. position of function   _____

10. range of motion   _____

11. sciatic nerve   _____

12. sensory nerve   _____

13. spontaneous reduction   _____

14. sprain   _____

15. traction   _____

Matching: Match each bone injury to its splinting procedure. Place the letter of the best procedure listed on the line in front of the injury.

1. _____ clavicle
2. _____ mid-lower arm
3. _____ wrist
4. _____ pelvis
5. _____ mid-upper leg
6. _____ patella
7. _____ ankle

a. flexible splint
b. traction splint
c. PASG/MAST
d. pillow splint
e. a pair of padded board splints
f. sling and swathe
g. rigid splint

True or False: Read each statement regarding splinting principles and decide if it is TRUE or FALSE. Place T or F on the line before each statement.

1. _____ Splinting an injury should take place immediately.
2. _____ It is best to manually stabilize a suspected fracture before applying any device.
3. _____ Place straps or cravats directly over the injured site.
4. _____ Control any bleeding before splinting.
5. _____ Evaluate pulses, movement, and sensation proximal to the injury.
6. _____ Check for weight-bearing ability before and after splinting.
7. _____ BSI is necessary when caring for an open fracture.
8. _____ Place padding into the spaces between limb and splint.
9. _____ Reassess the limb after splinting.
10. _____ Attempt to splint in position found.
11. _____ Expose the injured limb before splinting.
12. _____ Do not elevate an injured leg.
13. _____ Immobilize the joints above and below a suspected fracture.
14. _____ In a suspected dislocation, realign the joint if pulses are present.
15. _____ Loss of pulses after splinting may be due to tight bandages.

Fill in the Blank: Complete the following sentences on signs and symptoms of bone injuries by filling in the missing word or words.

Next to most _____ _____ lies an artery, a_____, and a _____. Surrounding the bone are muscles, _____, and soft tissues. Covering all of this is skin. If a broken bone end cuts an artery, there will be bleeding into the tissues, causing the area to become _____, _____, and _____. Disruption of an artery can cause loss of _____ distal to the injury.

If a sensory nerve is injured, the patient may complain of numbness or tingling, called _____. If the motor nerve has been injured, however, the EMT may see signs of weakness of movement or _____. If there is no movement of the extremity or _____, check the opposite extremity. Loss of movement on both sides should alert the EMT to possible _____ injury.

A grating sensation called _____ can often be noted when the patient moves an injured extremity. This is caused by bone ends _____ against each other. It is not necessary for the EMT to elicit this! Sudden pain at the exact location of the injury is called _____ _____.

During the general impression, the EMT may notice that the patient is protecting or self-splinting an injury. This is called _____.

Listing: List the 10 signs/symptoms of a suspected fracture.

1. _____
2. _____
3. _____
4. _____
5. _____
6. _____
7. _____
8. _____
9. _____
10. _____

Reviewing: List the word associated with each letter of the mnemonic for assessing injuries.

1. D _____
2. C _____
3. A _____
4. P _____
5. B _____
6. T _____
7. L _____
8. S _____

Short Answer: Answer each of the following questions from your reading.

1. Why must the EMT immobilize the joints above and below a suspected fracture site?

2. Why should the EMT splint a suspected dislocated joint in the position found?

3. Explain why a wilderness EMT may need to realign a dislocation before transporting the patient. Is this the same or different for an EMT functioning in a large city? Why?

Critical Thinking 1: Read this scenario and then answer the questions that follow.

Dan and Greg were called to the scene of a motorcross bike rally. There they found Michael, a 16-year-old who had injured his arm while fixing a bike. Michael was seated at the first-aid station, holding his left arm close to his body.

1. What do the EMTs know about Michael from this encounter?

Michael had caught his left forearm in a spring-loaded piece of equipment. A fellow biker had released the equipment, and assisted Michael to the first-aid station. There was no loss of consciousness or fall with this injury.

2. Describe the trauma assessment that Dan and Greg should follow in managing this situation.

The results of the assessment showed that Michael had a swollen, deformed, and painful left forearm. There was point tenderness at approximately the mid-forearm, and crepitus was noted when Michael tried to shift his arm. Michael could wiggle his fingers, feel touch to his hand, and there was a strong radial pulse felt.

3. Describe the management of this injury, including the splinting procedure.

4. Would Dan and Greg need to treat Michael differently if there was a laceration with bleeding observed over the area of point tenderness? If so, how?

5. How would the management change if there were no radial pulses noted on Michael's left arm?

Critical Thinking 2: Read this scenario and then answer the questions that follow.

Nora and Chris were called to the local high school for Brent, a center for the varsity basketball team. Brent had been playing hard when he could not bear weight on his right leg, and slumped to the floor in a seated position. He told the coach that it felt like his knee had given way, and that he could not move it. When Nora and Chris arrived, Brent was seated on the bench, splinting his knee, his right leg extended. Initial exam showed no life threats. The detailed trauma exam showed deformity to the right knee with swelling on the lateral aspect, inability to move the right leg, strong pedal pulse, and good sensation. The EMTs splinted the knee in the position found and transported Brent to the ED. They reported that Brent had a dislocated knee.

1. Do you agree or disagree with the assessment of a dislocated knee? If you disagree, what is the likely injury?

2. Do you agree or disagree with the management of Brent's injury? If you disagree, how would you manage the injury?

Student Name _____ Date _____

Skill 34–1: Application of the Bipolar Traction Splint

Purpose: To apply a traction device to a possible midshaft femur fracture.

Standard Precautions:
- Hand washing
- Gloves

Equipment Needed:

1. Bipolar traction splint

Yes: ❑   Reteach: ❑   Return: ❑   Instructor initials: _____

Step One: Apply manual stabilization of the limb, while instructing another trained assistant to grasp the leg just above the knee, applying manual stabilization of the affected leg.

Yes: ❑   Reteach: ❑   Return: ❑   Instructor initials: _____

Step Two: Check distal pulses, movement, and circulation in the affected leg.

Yes: ❑   Reteach: ❑   Return: ❑   Instructor initials: _____

Step Three: Prepare the traction device, adjust it beyond the length of the uninjured leg, and move the straps into place.

Yes: ❑   Reteach: ❑   Return: ❑   Instructor initials: _____

Step Four: Apply the ankle hitch to the ankle, and assume traction of the leg.

Yes: ❑   Reteach: ❑   Return: ❑   Instructor initials: _____

Step Five: Slide the traction splint under the legs, and secure the ischial strap across the thigh.

Yes: ❑   Reteach: ❑   Return: ❑   Instructor initials: _____

Step Six: In the last step, apply the ankle hitch to the ratchet and apply mechanical traction. With the straps in place, recheck distal pulses, movement, and sensation.

Yes: ❑   Reteach: ❑   Return: ❑   Instructor initials: _____

Student Name _____ Date _____

Skill 34–2: Application of a Unipolar Traction Splint

Purpose: To apply a traction device to a possible midshaft femur fracture.

Standard Precautions:
- Hand washing
- Gloves

Equipment Needed:

1. Scissors
2. Unipolar traction device

Yes: ❑   Reteach: ❑   Return: ❑   Instructor initials: _____

Step One: Apply manual stabilization of the limb, while instructing another trained assistant to grasp the leg just above the knee, in order to apply manual stabilization of the affected leg.

Yes: ❑   Reteach: ❑   Return: ❑   Instructor initials: _____

Step Two: Check distal pulses, movement, and circulation in the affected leg.

Yes: ❑   Reteach: ❑   Return: ❑   Instructor initials: _____

Step Three: Prepare the traction device, adjusting it about 3–4 inches past the leg.

Yes: ❑   Reteach: ❑   Return: ❑   Instructor initials: _____

Step Four: Slide the traction splint between the legs, and secure the ischial strap across the thigh.

Yes: ❑   Reteach: ❑   Return: ❑   Instructor initials: _____

Step Five: Apply the ankle hitch to the ankle, and apply traction of the leg.

Yes: ❑   Reteach: ❑   Return: ❑   Instructor initials: _____

Step Six: In the last step, place the straps in place, and recheck distal pulses, movement, and sensation.

Yes: ❑   Reteach: ❑   Return: ❑   Instructor initials: _____

189

CHAPTER 35 PRENATAL PROBLEMS

An EMT may be called to the scene of a woman who is having a complication of pregnancy. He now has two lives to consider, but prompt attention to life-threatening complications can help to ensure survival of both mother and child in many cases.

True or False: Read each sentence and determine if it is TRUE or FALSE. Write T or F on the line.

1. _____ A woman with abdominal pain should be suspected of having appendicitis.

2. _____ A pregnancy outside the uterus is called an ectopic pregnancy.

3. _____ Ectopic pregnancies pose the greatest risk to the mother at 9 months.

4. _____ The location of the ectopic pregnancy poses little risk of hemorrhage or shock.

5. _____ Hypotension is normal during an ectopic pregnancy.

6. _____ Vaginal bleeding during pregnancy should be considered serious.

7. _____ Premature separation of the placenta from the uterus is called a prolapse.

8. _____ Placenta previa is when the placenta grows over the cervix.

9. _____ Spontaneous abortions are also called miscarriages.

10. _____ Seat belts decrease maternal and infant mortality.

Identification: Read each definition and write the correct word or phrase after it.

1. Loss of a pregnancy _____

2. A convulsive disorder seen only in pregnancy _____

3. The afterbirth grows over the cervix _____

4. Compression of the vena cava with a drop in blood pressure when the pregnant woman lies flat _____

5. An inflammation of the appendix _____

6. Nonmedical term used to describe a loss of a pregnancy, usually early in the pregnancy _____

7. A pregnancy outside the uterus _____

8. The afterbirth prematurely dislodges from the uterine wall _____

Fill in the Blank: Complete each sentence by filling in the missing word or words.

Pregnancy changes the way the body takes care of itself. The pregnant woman's heart is normally _____ than the nonpregnant woman, and her blood pressure is usually_____. The EMT should remember that the pregnant woman has manufactured approximately _____% more blood than usual, and so a significant blood loss can occur before there is a change in _____ _____.

   The EMT must remember that in managing any trauma in pregnancy, he must concentrate on saving the _____.

Short Answer: Answer the following questions.

1. In addition to vital signs, what assessments should the EMT use in determining shock in the pregnant patient? Why?

2. Name at least three mechanisms of injury that are likely to cause trauma to the pregnant woman and fetus.

3. Why are pregnant women at risk for these mechanisms of injury?

Critical Thinking: Read the scenario and then answer the questions afterward.

The dispatcher had sent Denise and Steve to the Cassidy home for a "pregnancy related" problem. Upon their arrival, they found Mrs. Cassidy lying on the couch. She stated that she was 8 months pregnant, with the baby due in 4 weeks. That morning, while ironing, there was some bleeding from the vagina. The bleeding had increased, and she then called her doctor and 911.

1. List the assessments that the EMTs must make at this point.

Mrs. Cassidy told Steve that she did not have any pain with this bleeding, had not noticed any contractions, and did not injure herself.

2. What is the likely cause of Mrs. Cassidy's bleeding?

3. How should Steve and Denise manage Mrs. Cassidy?

CHAPTER 36 EMERGENCY CHILDBIRTH

Even though pregnancy is a common condition, childbirth rarely occurs in the field! Although EMTs do not often encounter this type of situation, they must familiarize themselves with and review the basic principles of childbirth.

Word Scramble: Unscramble the following words. Use the clues to help you.

1. Thinning of the cervix   mtffnaccee   _____
2. Process in which the fetus is expelled from the uterus   rolba   _____
3. Term to describe a woman who has had children   prsouaitlmu   _____
4. Term to describe a woman in her first pregnancy   soruapiirmp   _____
5. Appearance of the fetal head at the vagina   growncin   _____
6. Total number of pregnancies   vidarga   _____
7. Total number of live children born to a woman   raap   _____
8. Movement of the cranial bones in a delivering fetus   gomlind   _____
9. Fetal stool   nocmmuie   _____

Definitions: Write the definitions of the following Key Terms from Chapter 36 of the textbook.

1. amniotic sac   _____
   _____

2. cervical dilation   _____
   _____

3. bloody show   _____
   _____

4. Braxton Hicks contractions   _____
   _____

5. cardinal movements of labor   _____
   _____

6. prolapsed umbilical cord   _____
   _____

7. breach presentation   _____
   _____

8. premature delivery   _____
   _____

Sorting: Determine whether the description is of the first, second, or third stage of labor. Write the description under the correct stage.

effacement

delivery of the infant

rupture of the amniotic sac

delivery of the placenta

full cervical dilation

infant's head pushing on rectum

crowning

gushing of blood, approximately 250–500 cc

First stage   **Second stage**   **Third stage**

Identification: Place a check mark in front of the essential components of a predelivery history.

_____ Due date

_____ Blood pressure

_____ Any complications during the pregnancy

_____ Crowning

_____ Prenatal care

_____ Any fluids from the vagina

_____ Time when contractions started

_____ BSI

_____ Maternal weight

_____ How long each contraction lasts

_____ Gravida

_____ Parity

Sorting: Decide if the EMT should assist the mother to deliver in the field, or begin transport to the hospital. Put each situation under the likely location.

primiparous, contractions 10 minutes apart

crowning

irregular contractions

multiparous, contractions 2 minutes apart

need to move bowels

increased vaginal pressure

need to push

primiparous, regular contractions, no observation of fetal head

Field delivery   **Transport**

Listing: State the use for each component in the OB kit.

1. surgical scissors

2. clamps

3. bulb suction

4. towels

5. gauze sponges

6. BSI

7. blanket

8. plastic bag

Ordering: Place the following steps for a field delivery in order. Place a numeral 1 before the first step, a 2 before the second step, and so on.

_____ Deliver placenta

_____ Position the mother

_____ Gentle pressure on the infant's head during crowning

_____ Check for cord around the neck

_____ Record time and place of delivery

_____ Suction mouth and then nose of infant

_____ BSI

_____ Clamp cord when pulsations have stopped

_____ Dry infant and wrap

_____ Support the infant's weight during delivery

_____ Transport mother, infant, and placenta to hospital

Critical Thinking: Read the following scenario and then answer the questions afterwards.

Deb and Rhonda, both EMTs, arrived at the home of Grace Hayfield, a 22-year-old female. Grace was expecting her first child and believed that labor had begun. When Deb and Rhonda asked her due date, she told them the baby was not due for 4 weeks but she was having intense contractions every 4 minutes, and her water had broken. While Deb prepared to perform a discreet visual exam of the perineum, Rhonda asked about prenatal care. Grace confessed that she had never seen a doctor for the pregnancy because she did not have any insurance, and the baby's father was not willing to assist. Deb informed Rhonda that the infant's head was present at the vaginal opening, and delivery was imminent.

1. What equipment will Deb and Rhonda need for the field delivery?

2. What should the EMTs tell Grace regarding the plan of care?

3. Should the EMTs contact Medical Control? Why or why not?

The field delivery proceeded without a hitch; a beautiful baby girl who was breathing well on her own, crying loudly, and turning nice and pink. Deb said she would complete the newborn assessment while Rhonda prepared to deliver the placenta. Rhonda noted that Grace still appeared "very pregnant" and the placenta had not appeared.

4. What is the likely explanation for Grace's appearance?

5. What should the EMTs do now?

Student Name _____ Date _____

Skill 36–1: Emergency Delivery

Purpose: To assist the mother in the natural delivery of a new born infant.

Standard Precautions:
- Hand washing
- Gloves
- Gown
- Mask
- Goggles

Equipment Needed:

1. Surgical scissors or cord clamps
2. Bulb suction device
3. Towels
4. Gauze sponges
5. Baby blanket
6. Sanitary napkins
7. Plastic bag or bucket

Yes: ❏   Reteach: ❏   Return: ❏   Instructor initials: _____

Step One: Position the mother supine, with knees drawn up and spread apart, and assist by helping her to elevate her buttocks on a pillow or blankets.

Yes: ❏   Reteach: ❏   Return: ❏   Instructor initials: _____

Step Two: Create a clean area around the vaginal opening with clean towels or paper barriers.

Yes: ❏   Reteach: ❏   Return: ❏   Instructor initials: _____

Step Three: As the infant's head appears, during crowning, place fingers gently on the skull and exert very gentle pressure to prevent explosive delivery.

Yes: ❏   Reteach: ❏   Return: ❏   Instructor initials: _____

Step Four: If the amniotic sac has not broken, use thumb and forefinger, or a clamp, to puncture the sac and push it away from the infant's head and face.

Yes: ❏   Reteach: ❏   Return: ❏   Instructor initials: _____

(continues)

Skill 36–1: Continued

Step Five: As the infant's head is delivered, determine if the umbilical cord is around the neck; if it is, slip it over the infant's head or shoulder. If it is not possible to slip the cord, clamp the cord in two places, cut the cord between the clamps, and unwrap the cord from the infant's neck.

Yes: ❑   Reteach: ❑   Return: ❑   Instructor initials: _____

Step Six: After the infant's head is born, support the head, and suction the newborn's mouth, and then the nose, several times with the bulb suction device.

Yes: ❑   Reteach: ❑   Return: ❑   Instructor initials: _____

Step Seven: As the torso and full body are born, support the infant with both hands. As the feet are born, grasp them firmly.

Yes: ❑   Reteach: ❑   Return: ❑   Instructor initials: _____

Step Eight: After pulsations cease, clamp the umbilical cord in two places, with the closest clamp about four fingers' width away from the infant, and then cut the cord between the clamps.

Yes: ❑   Reteach: ❑   Return: ❑   Instructor initials: _____

Step Nine: Then gently dry the infant with towels, and wrap the infant in a warm blanket. Place the infant on his side, preferably with the head slightly lower than the trunk.

Yes: ❑   Reteach: ❑   Return: ❑   Instructor initials: _____

Step Ten: Another EMT should monitor the infant, and complete initial care of the newborn.

Yes: ❑   Reteach: ❑   Return: ❑   Instructor initials: _____

Step Eleven: Place a sterile sanitary napkin between the mother's legs and have her close her legs. Also, comfort the mother and monitor vital signs.

Yes: ❑   Reteach: ❑   Return: ❑   Instructor initials: _____

Step Twelve: While preparing the mother and infant for transport, watch for delivery of the placenta. When the placenta is delivered, wrap the placenta in a towel and place it in a plastic bag or container, transporting it to the hospital with the mother.

Yes: ❑   Reteach: ❑   Return: ❑   Instructor initials: _____

CHAPTER 37 NEWBORN CARE

Although most deliveries are without complications, an infant is at high risk for potentially fatal problems in the first hour of life.

True or False: Read each sentence and determine if it is TRUE or FALSE. Write T or F on the line.

1. _____ A newborn with hypoxia is usually tachycardic.

2. _____ Pad the shoulders to keep the infant's airway in neutral position.

3. _____ The EMT should suction the infant's airway for no longer than 3 seconds.

4. _____ The infant's tongue is smaller proportionally than the adult's.

5. _____ There is no exchange of drugs from mother to her unborn infant.

6. _____ Start chest compressions on a newborn with a heart rate below 60 beats per minute.

7. _____ The EMT should perform three compressions to each ventilation in infant CPR.

8. _____ Meconium is a white, cheesy material designed to protect the newborn.

9. _____ Acrocyanosis is a severe birth defect.

10. _____ The EMT can usually palpate only two fontanelles on the newborn.

Sorting: Place a check mark in front of the circumstances that can lead to hypothermia in the newborn. Suggest a way to correct those circumstances.

1. _____ suckling

2. _____ placing the newborn on a table

3. _____ positioning the newborn on mother's abdomen

4. _____ leaving baby's head uncovered to monitor fontanelles

5. _____ letting infant stay in amniotic fluid

6. _____ swaddling

Ordering: Place the following management techniques into the correct order. Place a numeral 1 before the first thing to be done, a 2 before the next, and so on.

_____ ALS drugs

_____ Blow-by oxygen

_____ Chest compressions

_____ Drying, warming, and positioning

_____ BVM

Fill in the Blank: Complete each sentence by filling in the missing word or words.

Measuring heart rate, respiratory effort, muscle tone, responses, and color in the newborn is determined through the use of the _____ score. It is completed at _____, and _____ minutes after birth. The EMT must also assess the newborn's airway. Place the newborn supine and slightly head down. Use a _____ _____ to clear the infant's _____. The newborn is an obligate _____ breather. Respirations must be adequate.

Crying is a good sign. Even though respirations are adequate, the infant may have blue hands and feet. This is called_____. A heart rate of less than _____ beats per minute means that the EMT must begin chest compressions. Once the initial assessment and APGAR is completed, begin a _____ medical assessment. Sometimes the infant's head may appear misshapen. This results from the birth and is called_____. The head shape will return to normal. The EMT must assess the _____ cord, which should appear bluish white. The EMT must take care to appear professional and nonjudgmental, as new parents "read" the expressions and behaviors of the caregivers.

Calculation: Calculate the APGAR for each of the following infants.

1. Infant is crying loudly, kicking, heart rate of 120 beats per minute, sneezing after suctioning with pink body and blue extremities

2. Infant is crying weakly, blue body and extremities, heart rate of 90, no reaction to suctioning, extended limbs

3. Infant is crying weakly, blue body and extremities, heart rate of 110, sneezing, and clenching arms and legs to body

4. Infant is not crying, body blue, limp extremities, heart rate of 80, no reaction to suction

5. Infant has pink trunk and extremities, coughing with suction, heart rate of 135, legs and arms held in fetal position unless extended by EMT, crying loudly

Short Answer: Answer the following questions.

1. State at least two reasons why it is important to suction the newborn's nostrils.

2. List four indicators of respiratory distress in the newborn.

Critical Thinking: Read the scenario and then answer the questions afterward.

Donna and Jarrett, both EMTs, responded to a call for a woman in labor. Upon their arrival at the residence, they were met at the walk by Gary, an on-duty police officer who was also an EMT. Gary informed Jarrett, the crew chief, that Gary could not ride into the hospital on the ambulance, but that he could assist in any way that Jarrett needed. When they entered the residence, they found that Johanna, a 24-year-old mother of one, had delivered a tiny infant in the bedroom. The infant was apneic, bradycardic at 70 beats per minute, and cyanotic. He was not crying and did not seem to respond at all. Johanna was lying on the bed, crying. Her color was normal, her skin was warm and moist, with minimal bleeding from the vagina. The placenta had not yet delivered.

1. What is the infant's APGAR?

2. Describe immediate care for the newborn.

3. What can the EMTs say to Johanna?

CHAPTER 38 PEDIATRIC MEDICAL CARE

Familiarity with techniques of pediatric assessment, and the common illnesses in each age group, can help the EMT to feel more comfortable when faced with an ill or injured child.

Word Scramble: Using your Key Terms found in Chapter 38 of the textbook, unscramble the following.

1. upcor   _____
2. mathas   _____
3. inemgtnisi   _____
4. gettolitipis _____
5. grebfinied   _____
6. noscittrear   _____
7. relibef   _____

Completion: Complete the following table of developmental considerations and vital signs.

Age	Respiratory rate	Heart rate	Systolic blood pressure
Newborn			
6 weeks			
6 months			
1 year			
3 years			
6 years			
10 years			
Teens			

True or False: Read each sentence and decide if it is TRUE or FALSE. Place T or F on line.

1. _____ Examine a painful extremity last.
2. _____ Newborns do not yet recognize their mothers.
3. _____ Never permit the mother to hold the infant during your exam.
4. _____ Infants usually double their birth weight by 5 months of age.
5. _____ The 8-month-old infant is usually afraid of strangers.
6. _____ A toe-to-head exam is less intimidating for the 10-month-old infant.
7. _____ Toddlers do not like to be separated from their parents.
8. _____ Ingestion of foreign bodies is a common problem for a newborn.
9. _____ Toddlers and preschoolers are at-risk for accidental burns.
10. _____ The EMT should always obtain a history from the parents, not the child.
11. _____ Body image is important to the teenaged patient.

12. _____ The greatest risk to a child with croup is a fever.

13. _____ The EMT should examine the mouth of a child who has a harsh, brassy cough.

14. _____ A simple cold can lead to difficulty breathing in a child.

15. _____ An increase in the respiratory rate is a sign of respiratory difficulty in a child.

Matching: Match the disease or disorder with its definition. Place the letter of the best definition on the line in front of the term.

1. _____ Group		a.	present at birth
2. _____ Epiglottitis		b.	inflammation of the lining of the brain
3. _____ asthma		c.	results from rapid rise in temperature
4. _____ SIDS		d.	lack of body water
5. _____ Meningitis		e.	marked by vomiting and diarrhea
6. _____ Febrile seizures		f.	bronchospasms and inflammation
7. _____ dehydration		g.	unexplained death of an infant
8. _____ Diabetes		h.	bacterial infection with swelling
9. _____ Gastroenteritis		i.	viral illness resulting in seal bark cough
10. _____ Congenital disorder		j.	Altered sugar metabolism

Correcting: The following statements are false. Replace the incorrect word or words and write the sentence as a true statement below.

1. The cause of SIDS is a <u>bacterial infection</u>.

2. SIDS rarely occurs in infants between the ages of <u>1 week and 6 months</u>.

3. SIDS usually occurs when the infant is <u>eating</u>.

4. <u>Larger</u> than normal birth weight babies are at increased risk for SIDS.

5. Full resuscitation is <u>not</u> done for SIDS.

6. SIDS <u>can</u> be prevented.

7. Parents can be informed of what was done for their child <u>at the hospital</u>.

8. EMTs caring for a SIDS child will <u>not</u> be stressed after the event.

Short Answer: Answer the following questions.

1. You are listening to the lungs of an otherwise healthy 2-year-old. He currently is having difficulty breathing. You hear air moving into the right lung, but not the left. Based on his age and his exam, what do think is the problem?

2. Both children and adults can develop the disease, epiglottitis. Why is this disease more dangerous to a child than an adult?

3. Is it important for the EMT to differentiate croup from epiglottitis? Why or why not?

4. What are the signs of hypoperfusion in children?

Critical Thinking 1: Read the scenario and answer the questions following it.

Beth and Troy arrived at the Smythe home for a sick infant. Mrs. Smythe met them at the door, crying. She said her 16-month-old had a fever that morning. She gave her a dose of children's Tylenol, and placed her down for a nap. Now the infant was weak, listless, and not completely awake. There was also a rash over her upper body and shoulders.

1. Is there a potentially life-threatening condition present?

2. Based on the limited information available, what BSI should be taken?

3. What care do the EMTs need to provide to Mrs. Smythe?

Critical Thinking 2: Read the scenario and answer the questions following it.

Brent and Heidi responded to a call for a child "choking." Upon their arrival, they found a 6-year-old coughing vigorously. He was yelling that he never liked lima beans and that they made him choke.

1. Is there a potentially life-threatening condition present?

2. Based on the limited information available, what do Heidi and Brent know about the child's airway.

CHAPTER 39 PEDIATRIC TRAUMA

One of the most anxiety-producing emergencies for an EMT is pediatric trauma. Fortunately, the majority of pediatric trauma care involves integrating a few new facts into an already developed skill set. With practice, an EMT can become as comfortable with pediatric trauma as with adult trauma care.

Fill in the Blank: Read each of the following and then fill in the term it defines.

1. _____ Required by law to report suspicion of abuse

2. _____ A machine providing artificial breathing

3. _____ A catheter to drain excessive fluid from the brain

4. _____ Surgically created hole in neck extending to trachea

5. _____ Emotional, physical, or sexual harm to a child

6. _____ Flexible tube placed into stomach for nutrition

7. _____ Rigid tube placed in tracheostomy to maintain airway

8. _____ A special intravenous tube left in place for long periods

Identification: For each age group, list at least three likely mechanisms of injury.

Toddler   _____

             _____

             _____

School-aged _____

             _____

             _____

Adolescent   _____

             _____

             _____

Assessments: For each phase of the initial assessment, list at least two results that should concern the EMT regarding the status of the child.

General impression

Mental status

Airway

Breathing

Circulation

Short Answer: From your reading, answer each of the following questions.

1. A toddler and his mother tumble off a set of bleachers. Why is the toddler more likely to suffer a head injury?

2. Why would an EMT elect to keep a child in his car seat following a motor vehicle collision?

3. A toddler has been burned as the result of a small fire. In addition to burns, what other concerns should the EMT have regarding this child?

4. Give at least three examples of cases in which the EMT should consider child abuse. What should the EMT do if he does suspect abuse?

5. Why should the EMT caring for a child with special needs pay greater attention to caregiver information regarding vital signs and activities than his reference material?

Identification: Read each scenario and determine if the child should be transported to a level one trauma center, or to a local hospital.

1. _____ A 3-year-old who fell from a 10 foot wall onto a paved driveway

2. _____ A 10-year-old with swollen, deformed, painful arm, with no punctures or lacerations from a skating injury

3. _____ A restrained 5-year-old in a low-speed, rear-end collision at the mall, seated mid back seat

4. _____ A 6-year-old who was struck in head by a soccer ball, with immediate loss of consciousness

5. _____ A 12-year-old struck in face by a baseball, profuse bleeding from nose and mouth

6. _____ A 14-year-old fell off a snowmobile and was dragged through woods

7. _____ A 3-year-old with knife wound to thigh, sustained tachycardia

8. _____ An 11-year-old boy who cannot move after diving into shallow end of pool

9. _____ A 7-year-old with a 25 cent piece-sized burn from a flaming marshmallow

10. _____ An 8-year-old with tree branch impaled in back

CHAPTER 40 GERIATRIC MEDICAL EMERGENCIES

As our bodies age, there are characteristic changes that leave us susceptible to particular disease processes. Geriatrics is the study of the diseases of the older adult.

Matching: Match the following conditions with the appropriate description. Place the letter of the correct description on the line.

1. _____ arthritis
2. _____ delirium
3. _____ dementia
4. _____ dysarthria
5. _____ elder abuse
6. _____ facial droop
7. _____ osteoporosis
8. _____ polypharmacy
9. _____ pronator drift
10. _____ stroke

a. acute change in level of consciousness
b. physical or emotional mistreatment of the elderly
c. progressive loss of calcium weakening the bones
d. a test of neurological function
e. injury to brain due to interruption in blood flow
f. multiple medications by a single patient
g. gradual decline in intellectual and mental function
h. one-sided facial muscle weakness
i. inflammation within the joints
j. difficulty speaking

Identification: For each system, list the common changes that occur as we age.

1. Visual

2. Hearing

3. Cardiovascular

4. Respiratory

5. Gastrointestinal

6. Genitourinary

7. Musculoskeletal

8. Integumentary

Fill in the Blank: Fill in the blanks regarding the disease presentations in the elderly.

In the elderly, a _____ attack may present itself atypically, without the classic complaint of chest pain. This is called a silent _____ _____.

While a stroke or _____ accident can occur at any age, they are more likely to occur in the elderly. The neurological changes that occur result from a disruption of _____ _____ to brain tissue. Because the damage is _____, the person will lose a part of his body function. The most common type of stroke is an _____ stroke resulting from a blockage of blood flow. The other type of stroke results from bleeding into brain tissue and is called a _____ stroke. The most common type of stroke results in damage to an area that allows movement of arms, legs, and face. Therefore, symptoms of a stroke include _____ of the arms and legs, and _____ speaking.

Listing: List five things that the EMT should assess on each patient suspected of having suffered a stroke.

1. _____

2. _____

3. _____

4. _____

5. _____

Short Answer: From your readings, answer the following.

1. What is the difference between delirium and dementia?

2. Why is it important for the EMT to make the distinction between the two conditions?

Critical Thinking: Read the following and then answer the questions.

Martha Wittakers called 911. A strange elderly woman had arrived at her doorstep, claiming to live there. Mrs. Wittakers had tried to find where she lived but the woman was adamant that it was right here. When the EMTs, Tony and Lisa, arrived, Mrs. Wittakers was being served tea in her own kitchen by the older woman.

1. What is the likely cause of the older woman's situation?

2. Name other causes that the EMTs should consider.

While the EMTs were trying to gather any information from the older woman, their radio cackled. "Be on the alert for a 78-year-old female, wandered from an Adult Day Service area on Vine and Wisteria Street." Lisa advised the dispatchers of their current situation and requested a police unit to assist. Police arrived with the son of the missing woman.

3. Should the EMTs simply release the elderly woman to the son? Why or why not?

4. What should they do first?

5. What explanation should they give to the son?

6. Describe optimal care for the elderly woman.

CHAPTER 41 ADVANCED DIRECTIVES

Advances in medicine have made it possible to delay death. As we struggle with this, patients have begun to assert their rights to determine the course of their life and death.

Definitions: Write the definition of each word or phrase in the space provided.

1. advanced directive

2. DNR order

3. health care proxy

4. living will

5. power of attorney

True or False: Read each sentence, and determine if it is TRUE or FALSE. Write T or F on the line.

1. _____ Efforts to express the patient's wishes before he becomes incapacitated are called terminal directives.

2. _____ A person who is physically disabled cannot legally make end-of-life decisions.

3. _____ A disease in which there is no medical hope is called terminal.

4. _____ A durable power of attorney enables another person to make decisions for someone unable to make them.

5. _____ The Patient Self-Determination Act of 1991 protects the rights of patients and physicians.

6. _____ Hospice care provides care to patients only when hospitalized.

7. _____ Supportive care designed to ease a patient's suffering is called resuscitative care.

8. _____ An out-of-hospital DNR provides a medical order to EMTs.

9. _____ An agent, designated by a health care proxy or power of attorney, is someone entrusted to make decisions on behalf of the patient.

10. _____ Implied consent assumes that a patient would want treatment if he were able to express himself.

Short Answer: Answer the following questions from your reading.

1. What legal principles govern both withholding CPR and beginning CPR on an unconscious patient?

2. What are the differences between the living will and power of attorney versus a do not resuscitate (DNR) and health care proxy?

Critical Thinking 1: Read the following scenario and answer the questions that follow.

Bob and Greg were on their first call together. It came early, only a few minutes after the shift began. They received dispatch information for an unresponsive elderly woman. When the EMTs arrived at the house, they were met by the granddaughter. She handed them an out-of-hospital DNR signed by the patient's physician. Through her tears, she said her grandmother was adamant about not doing anything but she (the granddaughter) just was not certain her grandmother was dead.

1. What care is required for the grandmother at this point?

2. What care does the granddaughter need?

Critical Thinking 2: Read the following scenario and answer the question that follows.

Ambulance 4 responded to a large, old home in the northern section of town. The call was for an elderly man, who had difficulty breathing. Upon their arrival, they found the man lying on the floor with several relatives around him. One young man was saying that a DNR order existed, but three other relatives yelled that the older man, their uncle, had changed his mind.

1. How should the EMTs respond to this situation?

CHAPTER 42 EMERGENCY VEHICLE OPERATIONS

In addition to the vast amount of medical knowledge that the new EMT will learn, he must also learn the basics of EMS operations.

Matching: Match the following conditions with their description. Place the letter of the correct description on the line.

1. _____ wave off
2. _____ panic stop
3. _____ rotor wash
4. _____ approach path
5. _____ landing zone
6. _____ flashback
7. _____ due regard
8. _____ shoreline
9. _____ sharps container
10. _____ right of way
11. _____ EVOC
12. _____ siren mode
13. _____ hot load
14. _____ spotter
15. _____ wigwags
16. _____ traffic

a. area intended for the helicopter to come down
b. respect and consideration for others
c. privilege of moving ahead of others on a roadway
d. receptacle for used needles
e. emergency vehicle operators course
f. wind created by cycling of helicopter blades
g. placing a patient aboard a running helicopter
h. emergency stop for unexpected obstacle
i. alternating headlights on an emergency vehicle
j. a person who assists the driver in backing up
k. crossing and uncrossing of arms to alert pilot
l. obstacle free area for helicopter to come in to land
m. electrical extension linking ambulance to building
n. strobes reflecting back into driver's eyes
o. characteristic patterns of sound alerting others to emergency

Definitions: Write the definition of the word or term in the space provided.

1. controlled intersection _____
2. yelp _____
3. LZ officer _____
4. covering the brake _____
5. surrounding area _____
6. emergency ambulances _____
7. four-second rule _____
8. emergency services vehicle _____
9. touchdown area _____
10. wail _____

Listing: List four considerations for personnel preparedness.

1. _____

2. _____

3. _____

4. _____

Listing: List six considerations for equipment readiness.

1. _____

2. _____

3. _____

4. _____

5. _____

6. _____

Listing: List at least ten items for the vehicle safety checklist.

1. _____

2. _____

3. _____

4. _____

5. _____

6. _____

7. _____

8. _____

9. _____

10. _____

Listing: List at least eight items that should be placed in the vehicle front compartment.

1. _____

2. _____

3. _____

4. _____

5. _____

6. _____

7. _____

8. _____

Descriptions: Describe each phase of the call by giving an example of activities in each.

1. Alarm and alert

2. Initial information

3. Departure

4. Driving

5. Arrival

6. On-scene actions

7. Transport to facility

8. Arrival at facility

9. Transfer of care

10. Preparation for next call

Critical Thinking: Read the following scenario and then answer the questions that follow.

"Car versus train" was the dispatch. Janie and Brad, EMTs with Response Rescue, both thought this would be a bad one. Upon their arrival, they saw a freight train stopped on the tracks about 50 feet past the intersection of the roadway and the tracks. The remains of a blue car were at the front left side of the train. The driver of the car was trapped but alive. He was talking to the engineer. Janie gathered a history of events, and called a report back to communications. Brad began the initial assessment. The train had been slow moving and had begun to brake almost 2 miles back. As such, it was close to stopping at the point of impact. For some unknown reason the driver had not left his car. Initial assessment revealed blunt injury to the chest and an open femur fracture; extrication would be lengthy. They decided to call for a helicopter to transport to the trauma center.

1. Do you agree with the decision to call the helicopter? Why or why not?

2. Describe how the LZ officer will assist in landing the helicopter.

CHAPTER 43 PUBLIC SAFETY INCIDENT MANAGEMENT

A response to a scene with multiple patients or unknown chemical exposures may be very stressful and confusing. It is the responsibility of the EMT to bring order to these situations.

Definitions: Write the definition of each Key Term in the space provided.

1. chain of command

2. command post

3. decontamination corridor

4. hot zone

5. material safety data sheets (MSDS)

6. multiple casualty incident (MCI)

7. NFPA 704 symbol

8. START triage system

9. placard

10. triage

Matching: Match each term with its definition.

1. _____ incident command
2. _____ EMS command
3. _____ public safety officer
4. _____ research officer
5. _____ safety officer
6. _____ staging officer
7. _____ transportation officer
8. _____ treatment officer
9. _____ triage officer
10. _____ operations level responder

a. personnel to stop HAZMAT spillage
b. decides urgency of patient's illnesses
c. has responsibility for an incident
d. in charge of organizing care of patients
e. gathers information about HAZMAT
f. has responsibility for EMS at incident
g. responsible for safety of all personnel
h. organizes pre- and hospital resources
i. reports state of affairs to the media
j. assembles and assigns duties to personnel

Identification: Assuming you have two ambulances on scene and another en route, mark each of the following as green, yellow, red, or black, according to the color triage tag you would assign.

1. _____ A 28-year-old female with abdominal cramps, who states she is pregnant

2. _____ A 34-year-old male limping, who says his right ankle hurts

3. _____ A 46-year-old male with a respiratory rate of 36, who is desperately looking for his inhaler

4. _____ A 20-year-old female with a painful and deformed left wrist

5. _____ A 77-year-old male with chest pain on a 10 out of 10 pain scale, with good respirations and pulse

6. _____ A 4-year-old female, who is still apneic, after a jaw thrust is initiated

7. _____ A 16-year-old with an amputated right leg, below the thigh, respirations of 24, who is without a radial pulse

8. _____ A 58-year-old male with a weak radial pulse, who can only breathe if his airway is held open

9. _____ A 36-year-old female with a possible dislocated shoulder, without a distal pulse

10. _____ A 90-year-old female in cardiac arrest

Ordering: Place the following events in the order in which they should occur at an incident. Put a numeral 1 before the first action, a 2 before the next, and so on.

_____ Warm zone is established with a decontamination corridor

_____ Hot zone is established

_____ HAZMAT team is dispatched

_____ The first unit arrives at the scene of a rolled over tanker truck

_____ Patients are extracted from the tanker

_____ Patients are decontaminated

_____ Patients are treated

_____ EMS command is established

_____ Patients are transported

_____ Ambulance is staged in the cold zone

Research: Using the *North American Emergency Response Guidebook*, find the name of each substance.

1. placard #2717

2. placard #1203

3. placard #1046

4. placard #1680

5. placard #1274

Using the *North American Emergency Response Guidebook*, find the placard number of each substance.

6. lithium

7. zinc nitrate

8. strychnine

9. oxygen

10. copper chloride

Using the *North American Emergency Response Guidebook*, find the first aid requirements for exposure to the following.

11. placard #2902

Critical Thinking 1: Read the following scenario and then answer the questions.

"Quality Ambulance Units 1, 2, and 3, respond to Highway 84 for reports of a tour bus off road. Multiple injuries. Time out 1600." Unit 2 arrived at scene first to find a full-sized tour bus overturned. Many people were milling about, and others were screaming or crying.

1. What is the role of Unit 2?

2. What sectors need assignment?

3. How can Unit 2 handle the arrival of the media (e.g., TV reporters)?

Critical Thinking 2: Read the following and then answer the questions.

Jean and Stephen answered a call for a truck struck by construction debris. Upon their approach, Jean saw a large tanker next to some huge steel girders. She told Stephen to stop the rig so she could get a better look. "Uh oh," she said, "It's leaking!"

1. List three ways that Jean and Stephen can find out what is in the truck.

2. Once a HAZMAT scene has been recognized, what must the first arriving units do?

3. List the zones, and who may enter.

213

CHAPTER 44 RESCUE OPERATIONS

A rescue is an attempt to help another person who is incapable of freeing himself from confinement or danger. In order for a rescue to take place, there must be a live patient.

Matching: Match the following terms with their definitions. Place the letter of the correct definition on the line.

1. _____ confined space
2. _____ cribbing
3. _____ flat water
4. _____ loaded bumpers
5. _____ P.F.D.
6. _____ roll the dash
7. _____ safety glass
8. _____ snag lines
9. _____ tempered glass
10. _____ undertow

a. the front of the car is pulled away
b. stays in one piece after being broken
c. powerful down-currents
d. used to stabilize a vehicle's frame
e. last line of swift water rescue
f. area with limited openings for entry or exit
g. a body without current
h. personal flotation device
i. hydraulic compression dangerous to EMS
j. designed to shatter into tiny fragments

Identification: Identify each of the following as related to water rescue (W), vehicle rescue (V), or both (B):

1. _____ Forcible entry
2. _____ Cribbing
3. _____ Flapping of the roof
4. _____ Nader pin
5. _____ Point of contact
6. _____ Throw bag
7. _____ Window punch
8. _____ Undertow
9. _____ Swift current
10. _____ High life hazard

Identification: For each of the following situations, identify a safety item that rescuers should use.

1. Body fluids
2. Loud noises
3. Sharp objects
4. Flying debris
5. Poor visibility
6. Flash and flame
7. Falling objects

Short Answer: Answer the following questions.

1. Describe how a shore-based rescue is established, for both swift and flat waters.

2. List the phases of a rescue.

3. What is the minimum personal protective equipment that an EMT should have when extricating a patient from a crashed motor vehicle?

Critical Thinking 1: Read the scenario and then answer the questions that follow.

A semi filled with sand, blew out its front tire, careened across two lanes of traffic on the bridge, and came to rest on its side against the guard rails; the cab hung over the street below.

1. What type of rescue will be necessary?

2. List at least three safety hazards.

Critical Thinking 2: Read the scenario and then answer the questions that follow.

A rowing shell was struck by a motorized racing boat, approximately 15 feet from shore.

1. What type of rescue will be necessary?

2. List at least three safety hazards.

Critical Thinking 3: Read the scenario and then answer the questions that follow.

Three college friends explored a set of caves on private property. One of the students became trapped in a narrow shaft.

1. What type of rescue will be necessary?

2. List at least three safety hazards.

CHAPTER 45 ADVANCED LIFE SUPPORT ASSIST SKILLS

There are some situations in which the EMT will call for assistance from advanced life support providers. In these circumstances, the EMT may be able to provide support to the ALS unit, if the EMT is familiar with common ALS procedures.

Definitions: Write the definition of the word or terms in the space provided.

1. laryngoscope _____

2. hyperventilation _____

3. cricoid pressure _____

4. 12-lead ECG _____

5. normal saline (NS) _____

6. D5W _____

7. macrodrip _____

8. lactated Ringer's solution (LR) _____

9. microdrip _____

10. preoxygenation _____

Ordering: Place the following steps of preparing IV tubing in the proper sequence by numbering them from 1 to 6.

_____ Check the solution for clarity and date.

_____ Remove the tab from the solution, and the cap from the drip chamber.

_____ Select IV tubing size, open the packaging, and close the roller clamp.

_____ Open the roller clamp and allow the fluid through the IV tubing.

_____ Put the tubing spike into the appropriate IV solution port on the IV bag.

_____ Hold the solution upright, and squeeze the chamber to fill the drip chamber halfway with fluid.

Short Answer: From your reading, answer each of the following questions.

1. List four key "Do Nots" with regard to handling sharps.

2. Describe at least three ways in which EMTs help an ALS provider intubate a patient successfully.

3. Name and locate correct placement of 12-lead electrodes on the diagram below.

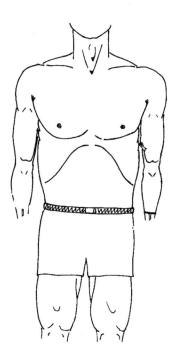

Student Name _____ Date _____

Skill 45–1: Intravenous Line Preparation

Purpose: To assist the advanced EMT by preparing the IV solution for administration.

Standard Precautions:
- Hand washing
- Gloves

Equipment Needed:

1. Intravenous fluid
2. Intravenous tubing

Yes: ❑   Reteach: ❑   Return: ❑   Instructor initials: _____

Step One: The EMT verifies that he has the right solution, the solution is not expired, and the solution is clear.

Yes: ❑   Reteach: ❑   Return: ❑   Instructor initials: _____

Step Two: The EMT selects the correct IV tubing, removing it from the box. He moves the roller clamp proximal to the drip chamber and closes the roller clamp.

Yes: ❑   Reteach: ❑   Return: ❑   Instructor initials: _____

Step Three: The EMT removes the tab from the solution, as well as removing the cap from the drip chamber end of tubing.

Yes: ❑   Reteach: ❑   Return: ❑   Instructor initials: _____

Step Four: Without touching either sterile end, the EMT inserts the tubing spike into the appropriate port on IV bag.

Yes: ❑   Reteach: ❑   Return: ❑   Instructor initials: _____

Step Five: With the bag spiked, the EMT holds the solution upright and squeezes the drip chamber to allow it to fill halfway with solution.

Yes: ❑   Reteach: ❑   Return: ❑   Instructor initials: _____

Step Six: Holding fluid up, with the tubing down, the EMT opens the flow regulator to allow fluid to fill the tubing slowly. Recap the sterile end once the IV tubing is flushed.

Yes: ❑   Reteach: ❑   Return: ❑   Instructor initials: _____

ANSWER KEY

Chapter 1

Matching:

1. c
2. g
3. j
4. i
5. f

6. e
7. h
8. a
9. d
10. b

True or False:

1. T
2. F
3. F
4. F
5. F

6. F
7. T
8. T
9. F
10. T

Short Answer:

1. Research has shown that trauma patients are best treated within one hour of their injuries. Prehospital care providers quickly remove trauma victims from the scene, assess and treat injuries during transport, and deliver the injured to trauma centers.
2. Military personnel were better trained to provide care to the injured, and had better equipment for field stabilization and rapid transport to definitive care at a field hospital. Their civilian counterparts had no standardized training, limited equipment, and most often used hearses or funeral-home-based ambulances for transports.
3. Johnny and Roy raised the expectations that Americans had for prehospital care.
4. Early Access, Early CPR, Early Defibrillation, Early Advanced Care
5. While EMT-Bs play a part in all four components, they play a direct role in early CPR and early defibrillation. EMT-Bs must be advocates for early access by promoting use of 911, and education regarding recognition and prevention of illnesses and injuries. In many areas of the country, EMT-Bs may actually be the provider requesting advanced level care.
6. Answers will vary.
7. Answers will vary.
8. Answers will vary.

Chapter 2

Ordering:

5	Assess patient	12	Replace any equipment used
8	Call medical control as needed	6	Move patient to the ambulance
7	Continue care during transport	9	Notify destination facility of patient
4	Determine mechanism of injury or nature of illness	3	Perform scene size-up
2	Drive safely to scene	10	Reassess patient
11	Give verbal and written reports to staff	1	Receive information from dispatch

Identification:

X	Airway maintenance	X	Hemorrhage control
X	Ventilation of patients	___	Suturing of wounds
___	Intubation of patients	X	Bandaging of wounds
X	CPR	X	Assisting in childbirth
X	Defibrillation by AED	___	Prescribing medications to patients
___	Manual cardioversion		

True or False:

1. T
2. F
3. F
4. T
5. F
6. F
7. F

Definitions:

1. certification: proof of satisfactory completion of a course of study
2. medical direction: advice provided by a physician or other higher medical authority
3. off-line medical control: physician involvement in protocol and procedural preparation
4. on-line medical control: direct communication between the EMT-B and physician while care is being given in the field
5. quality management: a continual process involving planning, execution, assessment, review, and improvement of the over all plan
6. professional conduct: behavior demonstrating a caring, confident, and courteous demeanor expected from all health care providers
7. quality improvement: actions taken to improve the quality of care given
8. prehospital health care team: multidisciplinary group composed of medical personnel, firefighters, police officers, and other health professionals that care for patients outside the hospital

Fill in the Blank:

1. classroom
2. clinical
3. hands on
4. classroom
5. clinical

Short Answer:

1. By reassuring bystanders, the EMT can reduce the likelihood of misunderstandings, and thus increase the safety for himself and his crew. Additionally, reassurance is a measure provided in an MD's office or hospital. Prehospital care patients and family/friends are entitled to the same level of care. Be careful not to violate the patient's confidentiality.
2. A clean, pressed uniform and clear name tag serve to identify the prehospital care provider. Patients are entitled to know who is caring for them. Also, this will ensure that the provider presents a professional attitude.
3. EMT-Bs must continually practice and update their knowledge and skills, as the field of prehospital emergency care is continually changing due to new research.

Critical Thinking 1:

1. The EMT-Bs have first violated the "Do No Harm" principle, as their conversation may be overheard by others, and can have an effect on their patient's personal life. They have also neglected to hold their patient's information in confidence.
2. Answers will vary.
3. The EMT Code of Ethics lists promoting health as a fundamental responsibility. This may include, but is not limited to, actions such as community health education, health fairs, and working with seniors or other community groups in promoting a healthful lifestyle.

Critical Thinking 2:

1. Planning, execution, assessment, review, and improvements
2. Retrospective quality assessment, and prospective quality assessment
3. Retrospective
4. Any answer related to the five elements in answer #1

Critical Thinking 3:

1. Assessment, administration of oxygen, assisting in the self-injection of a medication, transportation, and postcall evaluation
2. Following the directive to change the oxygen administration device
3. While the EMT-Bs are caring for the patient, they are acting as the physician's designated agent.

Chapter 3

Completion:

1. abandonment
2. confidentiality
3. evidence conscious
4. Good Samaritan Laws

5. Health care proxy
6. implied consent
7. legal duty to act
8. off-line
9. on-line

10. Bill of Rights
11. pattern of injury
12. restraint
13. causation of injury
14. standard

Identification:

1. expressed
2. expressed by parentis loco
3. implied
4. implied by emergency doctrine

5. implied
6. expressed
7. expressed
8. expressed by an emancipated minor

True or False:

1. F
2. F
3. T
4. F

5. F
6. T
7. F
8. F

Identification:

1. duty to act
2. a mistake
3. harm

4. causation of injury
5. a failure to meet standards

Yes or No:

1. NO
2. NO
3. YES
4. NO
5. NO

6. YES
7. NO
8. NO
9. NO
10. YES

Identification:

___ Leave all medical materials on scene
___ Turn off lights
_X_ Remember anything that must be moved for patient care
_X_ Do not touch weapons
_X_ Leave answering machines or caller identification devices alone

___ Cover the body to maintain modesty
_X_ Do not use sink to wash hands
___ Turn off TV, radio, and video equipment
_X_ Keep unnecessary people off the scene
Use the patient's telephone to avoid radio communications

Short Answer:

1. The patient must be: an adult, or legally considered to be one; competent; informed of the reasonable and foreseeable consequences of refusal; and have been offered care to the limit that he will accept and encouraged to seek further medical care.
2. By listening carefully, the EMT may hear or sense that the patient is fearful, or has not completely understood the information provided.

Critical Thinking 1:

1. Some states permit assessment and/or treatment for pregnancy or sexually transmitted disease based on the conclusion that providing such early care outweighs the parental right to consent.
2. Parent of a child, in the military, emancipated minor.

Critical Thinking 2:

1. The EMT-Bs need to listen carefully to what Mr. Rotelli is saying and not saying. They should then ask to begin with simple assessment and care, carefully explaining the need for each. They also need to advise Mr. Rotelli that his present condition may be a serious one, resulting in severe illness or death. If they are unable to convince Mr. Rotelli of the advisability of care and transport at this time, they must let him know that they will return at any time, and inform him of any additional medical care provisions in the community.
2. They should contact medical control for advice.

3. They need to document evidence of competence, informed refusal, offers of care to the limit Mr. Rotelli would accept, and the availability of care in the community, including their willingness to return.

Critical Thinking 3:
1. Begin CPR and contact medical control for guidance.

Critical Thinking 4:
1. Observe interactions between the parents and child. Also pay attention to both parents' and child's response to the EMT-Bs. Note the history given by the parents at different times and any history given by the child.
2. They should report observations only. They should not make judgments or draw conclusions. Report the child's physical condition, including injuries noted, treatment given, and the response to the treatment. Report the behaviors of the child and parents. Report all history given by the child and the parents.

Chapter 4

Fill in the Blank:

body substance	exercises
acute	casualty
burnout	flight or fight response
debriefing	chronic
lifestyle	unwind
survey	stress
stressors	techniques

Matching:

1. b	6. i
2. d	7. e
3. j	8. h
4. f	9. a
5. c	10. g

Sorting:

Physical		Behavioral
increased heart rate	muscle tension	avoidance
gastrointestinal distress	Emotional	withdrawal
anxiety	edgy	aggression
headaches	depression	procrastination
insomnia	irritability	alcohol abuse
fatigue	anger	drug abuse

Short Answer:
1. Prevention of a stressful situation means that the body will not need to physically respond by releasing hormones. Treatment afterward, while important, cannot undo the initial response to the stress hormones.
2. There may be many answers, including cross-training and rotation of assignments.

Critical Thinking 1:
1. Review the situation, including the activity in the ED at the time. Plan how and when to ask questions in the future.
2. Concentrate on goals.
3. Focus on the positives of the care given.
4. Find an aspect of the unit or its staff that is positive and helpful.
   (Many answers may be acceptable.)

Critical Thinking 2:
1. Yes. Even though this is a positive step, stress occurs from both positive (happy) or negative (sad) events.
2. Liz can try to concentrate on the goal she has achieved. She can focus on the warm wishes of her colleagues. She can begin to plan her practice as a paramedic.

Critical Thinking 3:

1. Long shift, many calls, physical and mental demands, stressed patients and families, pediatric calls, potential exposure to a disease, trauma, an ill child at home
2. Relaxation exercises, physical exercise, engaging in hobbies, travel, social activities

Critical Thinking 4:

1. Stress (physical complaints)
2. The inability of the EMT-B to prevent Mr. Linkowski's death is a significant stressor.
3. Many answers are acceptable. They should include a focus on the positive aspects of Mr. Linkowski's care, care offered to his family, and the steps the EMT-Bs took to make Mr. Linkowski comfortable.

Critical Thinking 5:

1. Joe is experiencing stress related to a previous incident.
2. Joe may experience physical, emotional, and behavioral symptoms/signs.

Chapter 5

Matching:

1. k
2. m
3. g
4. w
5. l
6. h
7. s
8. n
9. r
10. d
11. o
12. x
13. y
14. u
15. f
16. a
17. e
18. j
19. i
20. q
21. p
22. b
23. v
24. t
25. c

Integumentary System:

1. protects
2. epidermis
3. dermis
4. subcutaneous
5. appearance

Muscular System:

1. T
2. F
3. F
4. F
5. T

Skeletal System:

1. f
2. a
3. o
4. j
5. i
6. n
7. m
8. k
9. g
10. b
11. c
12. e
13. d
14. h
15. l

Labeling Figure 5–1:

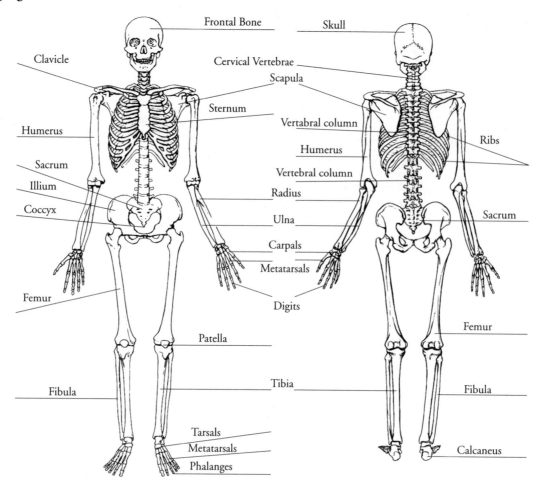

Frontal Bone
Skull
Clavicle
Cervical Vertebrae
Scapula
Sternum
Vertabral column
Humerus
Humerus
Vertebral column
Sacrum
Radius
Illium
Coccyx
Ulna
Sacrum
Carpals
Metatarsals
Femur
Ribs
Digits
Femur
Patella
Tibia
Fibula
Fibula
Tarsals
Metatarsals
Phalanges
Calcaneus

Fill in the Blank: Central Nervous System

The central nervous system is made up of the <u>BRAIN</u> and the <u>SPINAL CORD</u>. It is involved in the <u>INITIATION</u> and <u>TRANSMISSION</u> of all control messages in the body. The brain consists of the <u>CEREBRUM</u>, the <u>CEREBELLUM</u>, and the <u>BRAIN STEM</u>. The brain stem consists of the <u>MIDBRAIN</u>, <u>PONS</u>, and <u>MEDULLA</u>. The brain stem controls life sustaining functions such as <u>BREATHING</u> and <u>HEART BEAT</u>. The "athletic brain" is called the <u>CEREBELLUM</u>. The "athletic brain" controls <u>MUSCULAR COORDINATION</u>. The largest area of the brain, the seat of higher thinking, is called the <u>CERE-BRUM</u>. The brain is protected by three membranes called the <u>PIA MATER</u>, <u>ARACHNOID</u>, and the <u>DURA MATER</u>. The brain is also protected by a fluid called <u>CEREBROSPINAL FLUID</u>. The spinal cord begins at the <u>BASE</u> of the <u>SKULL</u>. The <u>PERIPHERAL NERVOUS SYSTEM</u> is made up of nerves that run from the spinal cord to take messages to the body. Automatic functions such as the heart beating are under control of the <u>AUTONOMIC NERVOUS SYSTEM</u>.

Labeling Figure 5–2:

A. ventricle
B. parietal lobe
C. midbrain
D. pons

E. cerebellum
F. medulla oblongata
G. spinal cord
H. skull

Fill in the Blank: Endocrine System

The <u>ENDOCRINE SYSTEM</u> produces <u>HORMONES</u>, which are chemicals designed to help the nervous system maintain control of the body. The chemicals are produced by organs called <u>GLANDS</u>, and are excreted into the <u>BLOODSTREAM</u>. They then affect <u>TARGET</u> organs to change the way the organs function. The pancreas is relevant to the <u>EMT-B</u> because it produces <u>INSULIN</u> that helps the body use <u>GLUCOSE</u>. Diabetics cannot produce this chemical.

True or False: Circulatory System

1. T
2. F

3. T
4. F

5.	F	8.	T
6.	T	9.	F
7.	F	10.	T

Fill in the Blank:

Beginning at the <u>RIGHT ATRIUM</u>, a drop of blood flows past the <u>TRICUSPID</u> valve and into the right <u>VENTRICLE</u>. From there it passes the <u>PULMONIC</u> valve, into the pulmonary <u>ARTERY</u>, and onto the lungs. Passing through the pulmonary circulation, the drop of blood returns to the left <u>ATRIUM</u> by the pulmonary <u>VEIN</u>. Moving through the left side of the heart, the blood passes the <u>MITRAL</u> valve into the left <u>VENTRICLE</u>, passes the <u>AORTIC</u> valve and into the <u>AORTA</u>, which is the largest artery in the body. This artery helps deliver blood to body tissues. Oxygen and nutrients are removed, and the blood returns to the right atrium via the <u>VENA CAVA</u>.

Labeling Figure 5–3:

A. apex
B. myocardium
C. purkinje fibers
D. interventricular spetum
E. superior vena cava
F. inferior vena cava

G. right atrium
H. tricuspid valve
I. right ventricle
J. pulmonary semilunar valve
K. left pulmonary artery
L. left pulmonary veins

M. left atrium
N. bicuspid valve or mitral valve
O. left ventricle
P. aortic semilunar valve
Q. aorta

Matching: Respiratory System

1.	l	9.	b
2.	j	10.	a
3.	n	11.	i
4.	o	12.	e
5.	k	13.	m
6.	h	14.	c
7.	f	15.	g
8.	d		

Labeling Figure 5–4:

A. oral cavity
B. nasal cavity
C. sinuses
D. pharynx
E. esophagus

F. larynx
G. cricoid cartilage
H. trachea
I. left lung
J. right lung

K. bronchi
L. bronchiole
M. alveoli

Digestive System
Fill in the Blank:

The beginning of digestion takes place in the <u>MOUTH</u>. There the teeth grind the food and allow it to be mixed with <u>SALIVA</u>, a digestive enzyme. The mass of moistened, chewed food is called a <u>BOLUS</u> and it passes the oropharynx and into the <u>ESOPHAGUS</u>, a muscular tube connected to the stomach. There, stomach <u>ACIDS</u> and other enzymes break the food apart. The stomach empties into the <u>SMALL</u> intestine where 90% of the digestion actually takes place. This intestine takes up the largest part of the abdominal cavity. Food then moves into the <u>LARGE</u> intestine, which terminates at the rectum. The rectum forms the feces, waste products, which are expelled through the anus.

Completion:

Organ	Type	Location	Function
liver	<u>SOLID</u>	<u>RIGHT UPPER QUADRANT</u>	detoxifies poisons
<u>GALL BLADDER</u>	hollow	<u>RIGHT UPPER QUADRANT</u>	stores bile
pancreas	<u>HOLLOW</u>	center	<u>HORMONES/ENZYMES</u>
appendix	<u>HOLLOW</u>	<u>RIGHT LOWER QUADRANT</u>	unknown
<u>KIDNEYS</u>	solid	retroperitoneal	<u>PRODUCES URINE</u>

Labeling Figure 5-5:

A. oral cavity
B. glands

C. pharynx
D. esophagus

E. liver
F. gallbladder

G. stomach   K. cecum   O. descending colon
H. pancreas   L. appendix   P. sigmoid colon
I. duodenum   M. ascending colon   Q. rectum
J. small intestine   N. large intestine

Matching: Reproductive System

1. h   7. k
2. f   8. i
3. d   9. b
4. g   10. j
5. e   11. a
6. c

Labeling for Figure 5-6a:

A. scrotum   F. ejaculatory duct
B. testis   G. prostate gland
C. epididymis   H. urethra
D. vas deferens   I. prepuce
E. seminal vesicle   J. glans penis

Labeling for Figure 5-6b:

A. ovary   E. uterine cavity
B. fimbriae of fallopian tube   F. cervix
C. fallopian tube   G. vagina
D. uterus

Chapter 6

Word Scramble:

1. immunization   6. immunocompromise
2. carrier   7. antibody
3. prophylaxis   8. microorganism
4. transmission   9. vector
5. contagious   10. biohazard

Listing:

A. Choose any five examples from pages 6–14 in your text.

B. 1. OSHA 1910.1030
   2. NFPA

True or False:

1. F   6. F
2. T   7. T
3. T   8. F
4. F   9. F
5. T   10. T

Definitions:

1. safety officer: a designated person in charge with knowledge of relevant CDC, OSHA, and NFPA regulations regarding safety
2. biohazard: refers to materials considered unsafe because of contamination with body fluids
3. personal protective equipment: gear that may be used by health care providers to protect against exposures or injury
4. immunocompromised: weakened immune state
5. infection control manual: document required of employers outlining risks, procedures, and care for exposures
6. risk profile: likelihood of presence of disease in a certain community

Identification:
X Ongoing health assessment of the EMT
___ Putting on gloves, gown, and mask before any patient encounter, and then removing what is unnecessary
X Carrying spare gloves for use with multiple patients
___ Washing hands only if gloves are unavailable or ripped
X Using goggles or safety glasses to protect the eyes
___ Putting on a mask only if you are close to a patient
X Using a gown for imminent childbirth
___ Using latex gloves for handling body fluids, and vinyl gloves for patient contact

Fill in the Blank:
The EMT should first put on FACE and EYE protection. He should then put on the GOWN if it is necessary. Assistance may be needed in TYING the STRINGS in back. Put the GLOVES on last. To remove the PPE, the EMT should go in REVERSE order. Remove the GLOVES. Then reach back and UNTIE or RIP the ties of the GOWN. Turn it inside out and roll it into a ball. Last remove the FACE MASK and EYE protection. Finally, WASH your hands.

Matching:
1. a
2. f
3. b
4. j
5. c
6. g
7. i
8. h
9. d
10. e

Sorting:
___ AIDS
___ tuberculosis
X hepatitis B
X rubella
X tetanus
X measles

Identification:
1. airborne
2. vehicle
3. contact
4. vehicle
5. vector
6. contact
7. contact
8. airborne

Short Answer:
In order for microorganisms to initiate disease, they must find a portal of entry. Hand washing flushes away microorganisms, preventing their entry into the body, or their spread to another person for entry.

Critical Thinking:
1. Remove gloves, wash her hands, and replace the gloves.
2. Use waterless soap or gel if a sink isn't available.
3. Provide any necessary first aid, and follow the *Infection Control Manual* for reporting the incident.
4. If any follow-up care is necessary, it can be started immediately. Also, should it be necessary, Jess's patient is present at the Emergency Department for further assessment.

Chapter 7

Matching:
1. f
2. h
3. a
4. g
5. j
6. i
7. b
8. e
9. c
10. d

Definitions:
1. ventilation: process of moving air in and out of the lungs
2. apnea: lack of breathing

3. cyanosis: bluish discoloration to the skin
4. epiglottis: cartilaginous structure at the base of the tongue
5. nasal flaring: widening of the nostrils during breathing; indicates respiratory distress, especially in pediatric patients
6. sputum: secretions from the airways
7. sublingual: under the tongue
8. gag reflex: protective response when the back of the throat is stimulated
9. occlusion: a blockage
10. Yankauer tip: rigid suction catheter with a curve and large open tip

Identification:

X	apnea	___	cough	___	conjunctiva
X	cyanosis	X	snoring	___	uvula
X	breathlessness	___	intact dentures	___	sneezing

Ordering:

_5_ Maintain open airway during entire call
_4_ Avoid pressure on underside of the jaw
_1_ Kneel at the level of the head
_3_ Push down on the forehead and lift up on the chin
_2_ Place the palm of one hand on the forehead and the fingertips on the jaw

Identification:

1. NPA
2. OPA
3. NPA
4. OPA
5. OPA
6. OPA
7. NPA

Correcting:

1. Suctioning removes debris and air.
2. Open, assess, suction, and secure the airway.
3. Suction to the depth of the measurement taken.
4. Adequate suctioning will take 15 seconds per attempt.
5. Apply suction while withdrawing the catheter.
6. Use a Yankauer catheter to suction blood.
7. French catheters are best for suctioning a tracheostomy.
8. Measure the depth of suctioning from the opening of the mouth to the angle of the jaw.
9. Flush catheters between each suction attempt.
10. It is necessary to wear gloves when suctioning. (Face mask and eyewear too!)

Critical Thinking:

1. They must have PPE, barrier devices, oxygen, suction, and airway-assistive devices.
2. Tania and Geoff should put on face mask, eye protection, and gloves.
3. Unconsciousness and snoring
4. Jaw thrust; no one saw what happened, and trauma cannot be ruled out.
5. Once the airway is opened, assess, suction, and secure.
6. An OPA must be done.
7. Geoff must continue to monitor the airway, as the body needs a continuous source of oxygen.

Chapter 8

Matching:

1. g		6. l		11. d
2. m		7. b		12. e
3. k		8. a		13. j
4. n		9. o		14. i
5. f		10. c		15. h

Identification:
1. Accessory muscles
2. Auscultate
3. Cricoid pressure
4. Intercostal muscles
5. Humidification
6. Dead space
7. Nasal cannula
8. Nonrebreather mask
9. Pursed lip breathing
10. Tracheostomy or stoma

Identification:
X seesaw breathing

X air hunger

X pursed lip breathing

__ cricoid pressure

__ apex

X accessory muscle use

X tripod

__ uvula

__ sneezing

Short Answer:
1. 21% oxygen
2. Moving a gas (air) in and out of the lungs
3. Adding or ensuring that oxygen is the gas moving in and out of the lungs
4. Yes. Another gas; for example, carbon monoxide, could move in and out of the lungs. Because it displaces oxygen, it would not help the patient.

Naming:
1. Pocket mask
2. Bag valve mask (BVM)
3. Flow-restricted oxygen-powered ventilation device (FROPVD)
4. Nonrebreather mask (NRB)
5. Trach mask
6. Humidification tubing
7. Nasal cannula (NC)

Short Answer:
1. There is increased flammability in the presence of oxygen.
2. Petroleum products may ignite.
3. Extreme temperatures cause pressure changes in the tank. This could cause an explosion.
4. Modified regulators may lead to leaks and they will fail to identify the gas in the cyclinder.
5. The tank may empty, leaving the patient at risk for hypoxia.
6. A tank may fall over. At least, it can injure a patient or EMT. If the neck of the tank breaks, it could explode.

Critical Thinking:
1. Posture, effort, accessory muscle use, mental status
2. Number of words spoken per breath, effort, patient's own description of problem
3. Tripod position, conservation of words, pursed lip breathing
4. They should assess the airway for patency, listen to the lungs, palpate the chest wall, observe any accessory muscle use, and assess the skin for color and condition. Additionally, they need an estimate of the breathing rate.
5. Ausculate
6. Mr. Allen is having respiratory distress.
7. Approximately 80–90%
8. Monitor for any changes, including a decrease in his level of response and the development of any secretions that may block the airway.
9. There is no need to place an assistive device at this time, but since Mr. Allen is awake, if one became needed, the EMTs could place an NPA first. They could change to an OPA if he lost consciousness.

Chapter 9

Identification:
X An unconscious patient in respiratory distress with an OPA in place

__ A patient who states that it hurts to breathe

X A pulseless and apneic patient

X An unresponsive patient who has taken an overdose of narcotics

__ A seizing patient with a paramedic expected to arrive in 5 minutes

__ A patient who is choking on meat but is coughing forcefully

__ A patient with facial injuries who has gagged on an OPA

X Driver in a car versus tree collision; CPR in progress

Matching:

1. k
2. f
3. m
4. l
5. b
6. h
7. e
8. a
9. g
10. d
11. i
12. n
13. j
14. c

Definitions:

1. pneumothorax: air in the pleural space, potentially causing collapse of the lung
2. hyperventilate: to breathe faster and deeper than usual
3. aspiration: a term meaning to draw into; refers to foreign material inadvertently being drawn into the airway during an inspiration
4. tension pneumothorax: air in the pleural space under tension, causing complete collapse of the affected lung and shift of the heart, and other intrathoracic structures
5. direct laryngoscopy: using a laryngoscope to directly visualize the airway structures
6. endotracheal intubation: placement of a plastic tube into the trachea

True or False:

1. F
2. T
3. T
4. F
5. F
6. T
7. F
8. F
9. F
10. T

Ordering:

1   Assess patient
8   Lift blade upward and visualize the cords
12 Ventilate and confirm placement
9   Place distal end of tube through the opening between the cords
13 Secure tube and reassess patient
4   Assemble and test equipment
3   Place OPA and hyperventilate the patient
10 Remove blade
7   Place blade into right side of patient's mouth and sweep the tongue left
2   Lubricate and place stylet
6   Place patient in sniffing position (provided there is no trauma)
5   Stop ventilation
11 Instill air into the pilot balloon and remove syringe

Short Answer:

1. Visualization means the operator actually watches the tube pass between the vocal cords.
2. In auscultation, the operator hears air movement over both lungs, but not over the epigastrum (stomach).
3. When an aspirator is used, air is easily withdrawn from the trachea, but not from the esophagus. Stomach contents may be withdrawn from the esophagus.
4. A CO_2 detector indicates pressure of the carbon dioxide produced during metabolism. It will register high on air from the lungs, but very low on air from the stomach.
5. When the tube is correctly placed, patient assessment will show improvement in skin color.

Short Answer:

1. The letters stand for those things that should be considered if the patient is not responding well after intubation.
   D   stands for displacement of tube.
   O   stands for obstruction of the tube.
   P   stands for pneumothorax.
   E   stands for equipment failure.
2. You should deflate the balloon, remove the tube, and continue BLS ventilation of the patient.
3. You should ensure the balloon is deflated, remove the tube, and continue BLS ventilation of the patient.
4. Pull the stylet back so it is one-half inch above the Murphy eye.
5. Deflate the balloon, pull the tube back slightly, reinflate the balloon, and reassess for breath sounds over both lungs.

Critical Thinking 1:
1. The EMT-Bs must begin with BLS airway and breathing maneuvers. Position the patient. Open, assess, suction, and secure the airway. Begin ventilation with a high concentration of oxygen.
2. Ensure that there was good chest rise with ventilations and continue.
3. Provide the paramedics with the reason for the EMS call, initial assessment, changes in the patient condition, BLS treatment, and the patient response.
4. The EMT-Bs must have oxygen, a BVM, and suction. If carried, they should also bring in the intubation equipment.

Critical Thinking 2:
1. They should perform a jaw thrust and then begin suctioning.
2. They need to perform all BLS airway skills, but also consider an endotracheal intubation.
3. Have another EMT hold stabilization of the head and neck, while the first EMT performs the intubation. Do not place the head in the sniffing position.

Chapter 10

Completion:
hemorrhagic shock

hypovolemia

PASG

stroke volume

decompensated

evisceration

irreversible shock

perfusion

urticaria

septic shock

cardiogenic shock

cardiac output

neurogenic shock

Fill in the Blank:
Starting at the heart, the blood enters the <u>AORTA</u>, the largest artery in the body. The aorta has many branches that serve head, chest, and abdomen. These branch further into smaller arteries called <u>ARTERIOLES</u>. These vessels contain <u>SMOOTH</u> muscle that allows the vessels to change their diameter. Individual cells are served by the smallest of vessels called <u>CAPILLARIES</u>. These smallest vessels and the surrounding tissues are the <u>CAPILLARY BEDS</u>.

Here, nutrients and oxygen are delivered to cells, and waste products are removed. Blood returns to the heart first by <u>VENULES</u>, then <u>VEINS</u>, and finally into the <u>VENA CAVA</u>, which returns deoxygenated blood to the heart. From there, the blood is sent to the lungs to be oxygenated and to begin another trip around the body.

Calculation:
1. 70 cc/beat × 80 beats per minute = 5600 cc/minute or 5.6 lpm
2. 70 cc/beat × 40 beats per minute = 2800 cc/minute or 4 lpm
3. 30 cc/beat × 130 beats per minute = 5200 cc/minute or 3.9 lpm
4. Patient #1
5. A maximal amount of blood is sent out from the heart. As long as ventilation and oxygenation is occurring in the lungs, the cells will receive more than enough oxygen per minute to meet their needs.
6. There was not enough time between each beat for the heart to refill.

Identification:
1. Hemorrhagic
2. Hypovolemic
3. Hypovolemic
4. Hypovolemic
5. Anaphylactic
6. Septic
7. Anaphylactic
8. Neurogenic
9. Cardiogenic

Ordering:
<u>3</u> brain

<u>2</u> abdominal organs

<u>1</u> skin, muscles, bones, and uterus

<u>4</u> heart and lungs

Identification:

1. compensated
2. decompensated
3. decompensated
4. compensated
5. compensated
6. compensated
7. compensated
8. decompensated

True or False:

1. F
2. T
3. F
4. F
5. T
6. F
7. T
8. F
9. T
10. F

Short Answer:

1. Anaphylactic, septic, neurogenic
2. Hypovolemia, hemorrhagic (a type of hypovolemic)
3. Cardiogenic
4. No, removal of PASG/MAST is based on volume replacement that the EMT cannot do.
5. Every 5 minutes

Critical Thinking 1:

1. Does Brittiany appear sick? What is her mental status? How is her respiratory status? What is her skin color? How long is capillary refill time?
2. This gives a good indication of Brittiany's mental status.
3. Children can compensate very well for decreased perfusion. By the time the BP drops in pediatric patients, shock is well advanced.
4. Supplemental oxygen, position the child flat, legs may be elevated as long as there are no contraindications, prevent heat loss, transport, call for ALS

Critical Thinking 2:

1. Tilt test, to check for orthostatic vital signs
2. Supplemental oxygen, position the patient in Trendelenburg as long as there are no contraindications, prevent heat loss, transport, call for ALS

Critical Thinking 3:

1. Hypotension (low BP)
2. Urticaria (hives)
3. Supplemental oxygen, position the patient in Trendelenburg as long as there are no contraindications, prevent heat loss, transport, call for ALS, and search for epinephrine prescribed for the patient. Do not delay transport to search extensively.

Chapter 11

Definitions:

1. anisocoria: unequal pupils
2. cyanosis: bluish skin
3. constricted: small/tight
4. jaundice: yellowish skin color
5. dilated: widened
6. pallor: pale skin color
7. diastolic: bottom number of the BP; reflects pressure in the vessels when the heart is at rest
8. PERRL: pupils equal, round, reactive to light
9. systolic: top number of the BP, reflects pressure when the heart contracts
10. sphygmomenometer: device to measure BP

Matching:

1. e
2. h
3. g
4. b

5. i
6. c
7. f

8. j
9. d
10. a

Calculation of respiratory rates

1. 30 breaths per minute
2. 20 breaths per minute

3. 24 breaths per minute
4. 12 breaths per minute

Calculation of pulse rates

1. 64 beats per minute
2. 90 beats per minute
3. 68 beats per minute

4. 90 beats per minute
5. 104 beats per minute

True or False:

1. F
2. T
3. F

4. T
5. F

Sorting:

Color	Temperature	Condition
pink	cool	sweaty
pallor	hot	dry
cyanosis	warm	
jaundice		
flushed		
gray		

Identification:

1. sign
2. symptom
3. symptom
4. sign
5. sign

6. sign
7. symptom
8. sign
9. sign
10. sign

11. symptom
12. symptom
13. sign
14. sign
15. symptom

Sorting:

S "difficulty breathing"
  tripod
  accessory muscle use
A eggs
M Ventolin
  vitamins
  aspirin
P lung disease
L breakfast this AM
  last used inhaler 1 hour ago
E smoker
  hot/humid

Chapter 12

Definitions:

1. firefighter's drag
2. rescuer assist
3. arm drag
4. pack strap carry
5. diamond stretcher carry
6. seat carry

7. end-to-end stretcher carry
8. caterpillar pass
9. squat lift
10. firefighter's carry
11. power lift
12. clothing drag

13. direct lift
14. emergency moves
15. direct carry
16. blanket drag
17. cradle carry
18. extremity carry

Matching:

1.	c	5.	f
2.	g	6.	a
3.	b	7.	d
4.	h	8.	e

Identification:

1. __ Person stuck in a car; complaining of leg pain
2. X Person unconscious from smoke in a fireworks factory
3. X Person with a fractured leg is lying across a patient in respiratory arrest
4. __ The driver of a car smashed his face and knocked out several teeth; airway patent
5. X Person is still inside a vehicle which has overturned into a creek
6. __ A person is complaining of back and leg pain
7. __ A person has bleeding from a head laceration
8. __ A person is complaining of mild shortness of breath following a fender bender
9. X A person collapses outside a building where there is a gas leak
10. X A person is in respiratory arrest following a minor accident

Short Answer:

1. Lumbar spine
2. Strengthening exercises for back and abdominal muscles
3. Squat down close to the tools. Pull them toward your body. Holding the tools close to your body, stand straight up using the large muscles of your legs. Do not bend or twist.
4. Use a draw sheet to pull the patient toward you onto the stretcher, or use a slide or transfer board.
5. Wearing the device tightly and at all times can lead to a weakening of the back muscles.

Critical Thinking:

1. Scoop stretcher or flexible stretcher can be used in the tight quarters.
2. An emergency move not requiring the use of the patient's arms. A clothing drag or blanket drag would work in this circumstance.
3. Any method that can keep Mrs. Hedderman sitting upright. The stair chair is safe and easy, but in a pinch, a chair carry would work. Ted and Katie must be assured of Mrs. Hedderman's safety if they use the chair carry.

Chapter 13

Completion:

1. The <u>INITIAL REPORT</u> is the first radio report of the scene conditions.
2. The feeling that there is an increased likelihood of injury is based on a(n) <u>HIGH INDEX of SUSPICION</u>.
3. A device intended to produce death is a(n) <u>DEADLY WEAPON</u>, while one capable of death or serious harm in certain circumstances is a(n) <u>DANGEROUS INSTRUMENT</u>.
4. The <u>PERIMETER</u> divides hazardous areas from nonhazardous areas. A barrier that protects EMTs and permits them to work is a(n) <u>SAFETY CORRIDOR</u>.
5. A scene <u>SURVEY</u> must be done to determine if any hazards are on-scene. Emergency vehicles can then be <u>STAGED</u> safely in a specific place.

Identification:

1. loaded, extent of damage
2. crumple zone
3. doors locked or jammed, windows open or broken, intrusion into body
4. cracks, starred
5. airbag deployment, mirror broken, seat belts used, wheel bent, headrest broken, cracked dash, pedals bent, seat knocked off pedestal, intrusion
6. fluids leaking

Identification:

__	Enter a car sitting on its roof	X	Turn off the engine	__	Close windows
X	Take the transmission out of drive	__	Chock the wheels	__	Cut seat belts
				X	Engage parking brake

True or False:

1. F	6. T
2. T	7. F
3. F	8. T
4. F	9. T
5. T	10. T

Correcting:

1. Replace "operations" with "incident command management"
2. Replace "scene survey" with "staging"
3. Replace "cannot" with "can"
4. Remove the words "two times"

Short Answer:

1. Broken rearview mirror   forehead
2. Bent steering wheel   torso
3. Broken dash   knees
4. Seat knocked off pedestal   body
5. Locked seat belt   torso

Critical Thinking 1:

The dry powder, spilled gas, angry patrons, curious onlookers, traffic

Critical Thinking 2:

High speed traffic, curiosity, loaded bumpers, antifreeze or fuel leaking onto ground, flares igniting fuels

Critical Thinking 3:

Poor lighting, lack of repairs, animals, guns

Chapter 14

Identification:

___	an injured, deformed leg		X	a stab wound to the chest
X	vomit in the mouth		X	absent radial pulse
___	history of a heart attack		___	allergy to penicillin
X	crepitus over the neck and chest		X	snoring respirations
___	a bone deformed in the arm		X	blood-soaked jeans
___	gives a complete medical history		___	breakfast last eaten
___	use of cocaine		X	tenderness of chest wall

Identification:

1.	alert	6.	alert
2.	unresponsive	7.	verbal
3.	verbal	8.	verbal
4.	responsive to pain	9.	responsive to pain
5.	alert		

Sorting:

Patent	Nonpatent
quiet breathing	snoring
speaking clearly	unresponsive
alert and oriented	vomitus
good chest rise	broken teeth in mouth
	infant unable to cry
	drooling
	stridor
	very bloody nose

True or False:

1.	F	7.	F
2.	T	8.	F
3.	T	9.	T
4.	T	10.	F
5.	T	11.	T
6.	T		

Definitions:
1. alert: awake and interacting with the environment
2. crepitus: the feeling of air under the skin; feels like Rice Krispies
3. sternal rub: rubbing the knuckles against the patient's sternum
4. flail chest: two or more ribs broken in two or more places, resulting in a free floating section of the ribcage
5. paradoxical motion: movement of the flail segment opposite to the rest of the chest wall
6. AVPU: acronym to remember the classes of mental status
7. ABCs: the technique of assessing airway, breathing, and circulation in order
8. unresponsive: cannot be aroused with verbal or painful stimuli

Short Answer:
1. The EMT can determine whether there is trauma or a medical complaint; whether the patient appears sick or not sick, and how fast the team should be moving.
2. The EMT must obtain information about rate and adequacy.
3. The EMT must control bleeding that is excessive in amount or potentially life threatening.

Determining Priority:
1. high priority
2. low priority
3. low priority
4. high priority
5. low priority
6. high priority
7. high priority
8. high priority
9. low priority

Critical Thinking 1:
1. The patient is unresponsive.
2. Since the patient is unresponsive, the EMT should presume that the airway is not patent.
3. Assign this patient high priority.

Critical Thinking 2:
1. No, there is not a potentially life-threatening condition present.
2. They know his airway is patent, and his breathing adequate for speech.
3. Assign this patient low priority.

Critical Thinking 3:
1. Yes; a complicated childbirth, and shock, are potentially life threatening.
2. They should anticipate that it will be inadequate.
3. Assign this patient high priority.

Chapter 15

Word Scramble:

abrasion	laceration
burn	puncture
contusion	swelling
deformity	tender
guarding	crepitus

True or False:

1. F
2. T
3. T
4. T
5. T
6. T
7. F
8. F
9. F
10. T

Listing:

1. Be polite
2. Give explanations
3. Maintain privacy
4. Make eye contact
5. Be honest
6. Focus the patient's attention

Identification:

X   Vehicle rollover with unrestrained patient
___   Fall of 10 feet
X   Death of another occupant in the vehicle
___   Farm trauma
___   Vehicle/pedestrian accident
X   Twenty inches of front-end damage
X   Ejection
___   Motorcycle accident
X   Crash speed of 20 mph or greater

Ordering:

5   Obtain baseline vitals signs
7   Document
1   Size-up/scene safety
6   Obtain a SAMPLE history
2   Complete an initial assessment, including spinal precautions
3   Consider ALS
4   Complete a rapid trauma assessment

Completion:

See Table 15-15 in text.
The acronym reminds the EMT-B to search for serious underlying injury.

Short Answer 1:

1. minor
2. size-up/scene safety; initial, focused trauma assessment; vital signs; SAMPLE

Short Answer 2:

1. major
2. size-up/scene safety; initial, rapid trauma assessment; vital signs; SAMPLE

Short Answer 3:

1. major
2. size-up/scene safety; initial, rapid trauma assessment; vital signs; SAMPLE

Short Answer 4:

1. minor
2. size-up/scene safety; initial, focused trauma assessment; vital signs; SAMPLE

Short Answer 5:

1. minor
2. size-up/scene safety; initial, focused trauma assessment; vital signs; SAMPLE

Chapter 16

Matching:

1. i
2. a
3. g
4. b
5. f
6. c
7. j
8. d
9. e
10. h

True or False:

1.	T	6.	F
2.	F	7.	T
3.	T	8.	F
4.	T	9.	F
5.	F	10.	T

Ordering:

_4_ rapid trauma exam   _5_ detailed exam
_2_ first impression   _3_ initial exam
_1_ scene survey/size-up

Listing:

Skull: DCAP-BTLS, plus extent of bleeding, remove glass shards
Ears: DCAP-BTLS, presence of drainage, Battle's sign
Eyes: DCAP-BTLS, raccoon eyes, size, shape and reaction to light, foreign material, accumulation of blood in the anterior chamber
Face: DCAP-BTLS
Nose: DCAP-BTLS, bleeding, CSF drainage, mucous drainage
Mouth: DCAP-BTLS, dentures or dental appliances, hoarseness to the voice, stability of teeth, bleeding
Neck: DCAP-BTLS, position of the trachea
Chest: DCAP-BTLS, crepitus, paradoxical motion, shallow breathing, lung sounds
Abdomen: DCAP-BTLS, distension, seat belt signs, urinary incontinence
Extremities: DCAP-BTLS, symmetry, pulses, movement, sensation

Critical Thinking 1:
1. Life threats
2. CSF drainage from the ears or nose; changes in pupil size, shape or responses; DCAP-BTLS of the head, neck, and back

Critical Thinking 2:
1. Abdominal distension, tenderness beneath the reddened areas
2. An abdominal injury with possible hypoperfusion

Chapter 17

Sorting:

S	headache	**P**	asthma
	shortness of breath		eczema
A	hives with penicillin	**L**	asthma attack 1 week ago
	wheezing after eating nuts		ate breakfast
M	Ventolin q6 hours	**E**	cleaning with bleach
	aspirin daily		
	Theodur QID		

Ordering:

_8_ ongoing assessment   _3_ OPQRST
_2_ chief complaint   _1_ initial assessment
_4_ SAMPLE   _7_ treat and transport
_6_ baseline vital signs   _5_ focused physical exam

Ordering:

_4_ SAMPLE history   _3_ baseline vital signs
_1_ initial assessment   _2_ rapid physical exam
_5_ treat and transport   _6_ ongoing assessment

Short Answer:

1. unresponsive medical
2. trauma insignificant mechanism
3. trauma significant mechanism
4. responsive medical
5. trauma insignificant mechanism
6. trauma significant mechanism
7. responsive medical
8. unresponsive medical
9. trauma significant mechanism
10. responsive medical

Definitions:

1. chief complaint: the patient's main problem, and the reason for calling
2. focused physical exam: physical exam focused upon the chief complaint
3. medic alert bracelet: a bracelet worn by those with chronic medical problems
4. ongoing assessment: the continued observation of the patient throughout contact
5. on-line medical control: speaking directly with the MD while caring for the patient
6. OPQRST: a device used to prompt questions related to the chief complaint
7. SAMPLE: a device to prompt questions regarding the patient's history
8. vial of life: plastic container with a listing of essential medical information

True or False:

1. T
2. F
3. T
4. T
5. T
6. F
7. F
8. T
9. F

Critical Thinking 1:

1. Medical alert jewelry, vial of life, family or bystanders
2. This patient would be considered a high priority, and transport should be initiated at the end of the initial assessment.

Critical Thinking 2:

1. The headache is the chief complaint; it is the reason for the EMS call.

Chapter 18

Short Answer:

1. Identify significant changes in the patient's condition, and evaluate effectiveness of care.
2. The ongoing assessment is begun after the patient has been thoroughly assessed, vital signs have been measured, and a transport decision has been made; also, the history and physical exams have been completed.

Identification:

X	mental status	X	empty oxygen tank	X	effectiveness of meds
X	airway	X	pulse oximetry	_	home safety
_	SAMPLE	X	distal pulses	_	abrasions to forearms
_	baseline vital signs	_	history	X	bleeding
X	breathing	X	pulses	X	pulse, respirations, BP

Critical Thinking:

1. Pulse has increased, mental status has changed, patient condition has deteriorated, priority is high
2. Respiratory rate has dropped, effort has decreased, patient condition has improved, priority remains high
3. Mental status has deteriorated, priority is high

Chapter 19

Definitions:

1. base station: original radio transmitters
2. communications center: dispatch
3. communication specialist: the dispatcher

4. med channel: ten frequencies used, nationwide, for communications between ambulances and physicians
5. tactical channel: frequency used for nondispatch communications
6. trunked line: system using computers to triage frequencies

Matching:

1.	g	6.	a	11.	f
2.	o	7.	l	12.	i
3.	h	8.	k	13.	e
4.	n	9.	b	14.	j
5.	m	10.	c	15.	d

Listing:

1. telephone interrogation
2. triage
3. dispatch
4. logistics
5. resource networking
6. prearrival instructions

Identification:

1. two-way radio
2. base station
3. mobile radio
4. repeater
5. portable radio
6. simplex
7. duplex

Sorting:

B	unit identifier	B	age/gender
B	ETA	B	chief complaint
B	mental status	B	vital signs
B	treatments in progress	C	SAMPLE
C	exam findings	C	changes after treatments

Short Answer:

1. They are able to prioritize 911 calls in order to only send units with red lights and siren when absolutely necessary. They are also able to give callers instructions over the telephone, with regards to medical emergencies.
2. Prioritizing of 911 calls, telephone assistance, and prearrival instructions
3. They are able to give medical assistance via the telephone.
4. The FCC regulates all communications and radio usage throughout the country.

Critical Thinking:

Alert Report:

Medical Center, this is Action Rescue Squad 1.

En route to your facility with a 70-year-old female who is complaining of a headache.

Vital signs are: respirations 16 and nonlabored, pulse 64 and regular, BP 198/98

We have the patient on high-flow oxygen and have requested an ALS intercept.

ETA is 20 minutes.

Consultation Report:

Medical Center, this is BLS Action Rescue Squad 1.

En route to your facility with a 70-year-old female who is complaining of a headache.

Neighbors indicate that the patient is not acting right today, although was all right last evening.

Patient is unable to answer to simple questions. She has no known allergies, is taking medication for a history of high blood pressure and glaucoma, and also takes an aspirin daily.

We cannot determine compliance with medications or time of last meal.

Patient is alert on AVPU scale.

Vital signs are: respirations 16 and nonlabored, pulse 64 and regular, BP 198/98

There is a droop to her mouth when she smiles, and left-hand grasp is much weaker than the right.

We have the patient on high-flow oxygen and have requested an ALS intercept.

There has been no change in patient complaint or condition since applying the oxygen.

Our ETA is 20 minutes.

Chapter 20

Definitions:

1. abandonment: leaving a patient's side prior to the completion of care
2. confidentiality: keeping conversations regarding patient information at a professional status
3. repetitive persistence: rephrase the same statement over and over again, until the patient understands
4. verbal report: a report given to the bedside nurse, or a doctor or nurse over the radio

Listing:

Critical Thinking 1:

1. She is not a nurse, she doesn't work at the hospital, and she is not the nurse for that patient.
2. Introduce himself to the person; ask whom to give report to.

1. Person
2. Place
3. Time

Critical Thinking 2:

1. Make eye contact, ask the nurse directly if she needs any further information regarding the patient.

Critical Thinking 3:

1. The patient can describe his condition more clearly; the nurse would prefer first-hand information.
2. All information included in the medical report should be given to the nurse at the time of patient turnover.

Chapter 21

True or False:

1. T
2. T
3. T
4. F
5. F
6. F
7. T
8. F

Fill in the Blank:

1. affadavit
2. objective
3. plan
4. subjective observation
5. objective
6. subjective
7. objective
8. special incident report

Listing:

1. Quality improvement
2. Legal document
3. Ambulance corps and/or state records
4. Research

Short Answer:

1. The closed format PCR has check-off boxes or bubbles for the EMT to fill. Patient information must conform to the boxes or bubbles. The open format allows the EMT to document observations in longhand.
2. It is useful for large quantities of data.
3. It allows for individual documentation.

Critical Thinking:

SOAP

S   C/C hurts to breathe

Patient states the motor vehicle collision occurred due to cell phone distraction

Allergy to penicillin
Takes a pill for high blood pressure
Has history of high blood pressure
Had hernia surgery 3 years ago
Just finished lunch
Denies loss of consciousness

O   40 mph posted speed
No skid marks observed
Restrained driver and only occupant
Steering wheel intact
Airbag deployed
A on AVPU
Speaking in 2–3 words per breath
Respirations 26 per minute and shallow

Tenderness over chest wall
Lung sounds clear
Vital signs BP 116/76 and pulse 100 and regular
Motor, sensory, and circulation intact

A   Shortness of breath
Chest trauma
Potential C-spine injury

P   C-spine stabilization
C-collar
High-flow oxygen
Short spine board to long spine board
Transport to trauma center
Reassess after movement and q5 minutes during transport

CHEATED
C   "Hurts to breathe"
H   Restrained driver, single occupant, struck tree
     40 mph posted speed
     No skid marks noted
     No steering wheel deformity
     Positive airbag deployment
     S   Grimace
         Shallow breathing
         2–3 words per breath
     A   Penicillin
     M BP pill
     P   High blood pressure
         Hernia surgery 3 years ago
     L   Lunch just prior to event
     E   Motor vehicle collision due to cell phone use per patient
E   A on AVPU
     Airway clear
     Lung sounds clear

Positive distal pulses
No apparent bleeding
Chest wall tenderness without deformity
Speaking 2–3 words per breath
No deformities of arms or legs
Motor, sensory, and circulation intact

A   Shortness of breath
Chest trauma
Potential C-spine injury

T   C-spine stabilization
C-collar
High-flow oxygen
Short spine board to long spine board

E   Motor, sensory, and circulation after move
Ongoing assessment q5 minutes

D   transport to trauma center
(turn over comments here)

Chapter 22

Identification:

1. contraindication
2. bronchodilators
3. protocols
4. actions
5. dose
6. expiration date
7. off-line medical control
8. side effects
9. indication
10. standing orders

Identification:

___	ventolin	_X_	pseudoephedrine	_X_	acetaminophen
_X_	ibuprofen	___	sudafed	___	motrin
___	advil	_X_	albuterol	___	tylenol

True or False:

1. F
2. T
3. F
4. T
5. F
6. F
7. T
8. F

Naming:
1. tablet
2. gel
3. suspension
4. nebulizer
5. gas

Naming:
1. IV
2. PO
3. SQ
4. IM
5. inhalation
6. SL

Listing:
1. right patient
2. medication
3. right route
4. right dose
5. right date

Fill in the Blank:
The EMT-B must <u>ASSESS</u> the patient and include physical and historical information on the patient care record. List the exact <u>NAME</u> of the drug, the <u>DOSE</u>, or how much was given, and the <u>ROUTE</u>, or the way it was given. Within 5 minutes of giving the medication, a <u>REASSESSMENT</u> of the patient should be done and findings from this should be included on the patient care record. Be sure to evaluate the signs or symptoms that led to the use of the medication originally.

Completion:
See text, and review Med Notes for each drug listed.

Critical Thinking 1:
1. albuterol
2. he had shortness of breath, a history of albuterol usage, wheezing in lungs
3. lung sounds, pt's ability to breathe

Critical Thinking 2:
1. EpiPen
2. wheezing, possible anaphylaxis
3. lung sounds, area affected with rash or swelling

Critical Thinking 3:
1. nitro
2. chest pressure, shortness of breath
3. chest pain, shortness of breath

Chapter 23

Word Scramble:
1. asthma
2. bronchospasm
3. crackles
4. croup
5. cyanosis
6. diffusion
7. dyspnea
8. epiglottitis
9. rhonchi
10. wheezing

Fill in the Blank:
1. accessory muscles of respiration
2. alveolar pulmonary gas exchange
3. cellular respiration
4. chronic obstructive pulmonary disease
5. congestive heart failure
6. hypoxic drive
7. pulmonary embolus
8. respiration, ventilation

Sorting:

Pediatric	Adult	Both
very flexible trachea	12-20 breaths per minute	wheezing
easily obstructed by slight swelling		
floppy large epiglottis		
tongue takes up most of mouth		
15–30 breaths per minute		

Matching:

1. c
2. d
3. e
4. g
5. f
6. b
7. a

Short Answer:

1. Pulmonary embolus: any from Table 23-1
2. COPD: cigarette smoking
3. Asthma: exercise, inhalants, cold, animal dander
4. Croup: child, upper respiratory infection
5. Epiglottitis: child

Completion:

Generic Name	albuterol
Trade name	Ventolin, Proventil
Indication	Signs and symptoms of respiratory distress
	As prescribed by MD
Contrainidication	Nonalert patient
Dose	Two puffs 1 minute apart
Route	Inhaled

Labeling

See Figure 23-1 in your text.

Short Answer:

1. Chronically high carbon dioxide levels cause the body to get used to the levels. The stimulus to breathe then becomes a low oxygen level.
2. Hypoperfusion is an acute event, the body does not have time to get used to it and switch over.

Critical Thinking 1:

1. Air passing through bronchioles narrowed by bronchospasm produces a musical or whistling sound called wheezing. In an asthma attack, some irritant causes the bronchospasm.
2. The reduction in wheezing meant that less and less air was moving through Kara's lower airways.
3. Diane must begin ventilation by bag valve mask. An ALS intercept should be requested if not already done so.

Critical Thinking 2:

1. Irritation of the larynx produces the characteristic barking cough.
2. Croup and epiglottis are often difficult to tell apart. The EMT should not examine Adam's mouth, as this could cause further swelling in the tissues and precipitate complete airway obstruction.

Critical Thinking 3:

1. Yes. Even though Mr. Williamson may be breathing based on hypoxic drive, he is currently having difficulty, and therefore oxygen should not be withheld.
2. Since cold air may further narrow his airways, the EMTs should be sure that he is adequately bundled up.

Chapter 24

Definitions:

1. angina
2. plaques
3. JVD
4. hypertension

5. thrombus
6. coronary
7. cardiogenic
8. myocardium
9. clot
10. tachycardia

11. diaphoretic
12. epigastrium
13. bradycardia
14. perfusion

Identification:

Modifiable: smoking, drugs, lack of exercise, diet
Nonmodifiable: sex, age, family history, hypertension, race, diabetes

Labeling:

See Figure 24-1 in your text.

Identification:

1. substernal chest pain
2. lower jaw pain
3. epigastric discomfort
4. shortness of breath
5. sudden weakness

6. shortness of breath
7. weakness
8. substernal chest pain
9. left arm pain
10. epigastric discomfort

True or False:

1. F
2. T
3. T
4. F
5. F

6. F
7. T
8. T
9. T
10. T

Ordering:

<u>8</u> complete a focused physical exam
<u>3</u> assess the airway
<u>6</u> obtain baseline vital signs
<u>7</u> get a SAMPLE history
<u>1</u> survey the scene for safety

<u>5</u> check circulation
<u>2</u> note general impression
<u>4</u> assess breathing adequacy

Short Answer:

1. Prompt recognition and treatment is the key to survival.
2. The heart muscle obtains its oxygen and nutrients from the coronary arteries
3. The treatment for each is the same, so it is not essential for an EMT to make the distinction. The recognition of a possibility of an MI based on risk factors and history, plus appropriate treatment, is the important point.

Critical Thinking:

1. Past medical history using SAMPLE
   History of this illness using OPQRST
   Focused physical exam including assessment of jugular venous distention, breath sounds, vital signs, pulse oximetry, and pupils
2. They must reassess for relief from the medication and complete the components of the initial assessment and vital signs.
3. Be sure Mr. Stevens is lying down and has high-flow oxygen. They should have called for ALS intervention and can contact Medical Control for additional assistance.

Chapter 25

Definitions:

1. defibrillation: application of an electrical shock to the heart in ventricular fibrillation
2. dysrythmia: any disruption of the normal sinus rhythm
3. electrocardiogram: the heart's electrical flow graphically displayed on paper or oscilloscope
4. automaticity: ability of the myocardium to self-pace

5. rhythm: regularly repeating ECG pattern
6. sudden cardiac death: unexpected cessation of heartbeat within 2 hours of the onset of chest pain
7. chain of survival: important steps that must be taken to improve cardiac arrest survival
8. public access defibrillation: public training in the use of an AED
9. artificial pacemaker: a man-made device that will create a spark, signaling the heart to beat
10. all clear command: an order that nothing should touch the patient

Labeling:
See Figure 25-7 in your text.

Identification:
1. asystole
2. sinus rhythm with PVCs
3. ventricular fibrillations
4. ventricular tachycardia

Ordering:
_3_ Open airway
_1_ BSI/scene safety
_5_ Check for carotid pulse
_4_ Observe for chest rise
_2_ Check responsiveness

Ordering:
_3_ Turn on AED and stop touching the patient
_7_ Reanalyze/reassess
_4_ Analyze rhythm
_1_ Assess patient
_2_ Apply patches/cable
_5_ Clear patient for shock
_6_ Press "shock" button

Identification
1. contraindication
2. contraindication
3. indication
4. contraindication
5. indication
6. contraindication
7. contraindication
8. contraindication
9. contraindication
10. indication

True or False:
1. F
2. T
3. F
4. F
5. T
6. F
7. T
8. T
9. T
10. T
11. T
12. F

Short Answer:
1. The usual cause of arrest in infants is respiratory in origin not cardiac. Efforts are best spent trying to correct the respiratory problem.
2. The EMT will need to provide care and support to the survivors.

Critical Thinking 1:
1. One of the EMTs should obtain the AED, while the other assesses the patient and the performance of CPR.
2. Once the patient has been confirmed as unresponsive, pulseless, and apneic, the EMT should apply the patches, turn on the AED, clear the patient for analysis, analyze the rhythm, and if shock is advised, clear the patient and press the shock button. If no shock is advised they should continue CPR, prepare for transport and call for ALS.
3. They should reassess the patient. If there is no pulse, continue CPR, prepare for transport, and contact ALS. If a pulse is present, they must assess adequacy of breathing, obtain vital signs, and prepare to transport.
4. The EMTs or paramedics should provide explanation and support to Mr. Roberts' family.

Critical Thinking 2:
1. The AED is to be used on patients that are unresponsive, pulseless, and apneic. The patient does not meet this criteria.
2. The EMT supervisor should tell Bev and Joe that it would be better if they didn't apply the patches just yet. He could offer to assist with further care and packaging. After the call is complete, the supervisor will need to review the standards of AED use with Bev and Joe. The EMTs may need to complete an AED refresher course of study.

Chapter 26

Matching:

1. n	6. e	11. o
2. l	7. j	12. m
3. k	8. f	13. a
4. h	9. c	14. d
5. g	10. b	15. i

Correcting:
1. A person experiencing a change in behavior that may be due to illness or injury is having a <u>behavioral</u> crisis.
2. A failure to remember what just happened is called <u>amnesia</u>.
3. Hypoglycemia is a lack of <u>sugar</u> in the blood.
4. Diabetes Mellitus occurs when the <u>pancreas</u> fails to produce sufficient insulin.
5. Excessive <u>urination</u> is called polyuria.
6. The development of <u>hypoglycemia</u> is a short-term event, often occuring over minutes to hours.
7. When the body cannot use sugar for energy, it uses <u>fat</u> instead.
8. Kussmaul's respirations are <u>fast and deep</u>.
9. Insulin shock results from <u>low sugar</u> in the blood.
10. A patient experiencing a low blood sugar will have <u>cool, moist skin</u>.
11. The cause of epilepsy is <u>not</u> well defined.
12. In a seziure affecting the whole brain, the <u>full body</u> is affected.
13. An <u>aura</u> is an odor or flash of light or sound that precedes certain seizures.
14. The post-ictal phase of a seizure occurs <u>after the body has seized</u>.
15. Managing a seizing patient includes <u>isolating the body from hazards</u>.

Short Answer:
1. The brain malfunctions when glucose is not available because it is the primary source of energy for the body.
2. They can still produce insulin; however, they may not produce enough to balance their diet.
3. Epilepsy is a disease of the electrical conduction throughout the brain. Seizures can also be caused by trauma or illnesses.
4. Patients can have a partial seizure and still remain standing. It would appear that they were "daydreaming" or lost the ability to speak

Critical Thinking 1:
1. It may have been caused by low blood sugar.
2. They should follow the ABCs and call for ALS.
3. Oral glucose is contraindicated, because the patient is unconscious and unresponsive.

Critical Thinking 2:
1. Head trauma from a fall may have caused this condition.
2. The EMTs should isolate the patient from any potential hazards and then attempt to protect and stabilize the head, neck, and spine.
3. C-spine precautions and ABC management should be the EMT's first priority.
4. No, because the patient is not conscious.
5. Yes, oxygen is indicated, because the child is unconscious.

Chapter 27

Matching:

1. i	6. f
2. g	7. o
3. d	8. c
4. j	9. b
5. h	10. a

Identification:

1. tactile	3. visual
2. command	4. auditory

| 5. auditory | 7. tactile |
| 6. command | 8. visual |

Identification:

1. extremity	6. positional asphyxia
2. extremity	7. four people
3. total body	8. show of force
4. papoose	9. medically necessary
5. takedown	

Sorting:

1. __ A young mother is crying after the death of her infant.
2. X A teenager is threatening to shoot himself after getting a bad grade.
   Request police assistance for safety. Once the scene is safe, be supportive but decisive.
3. X A young man is crying loudly after he dropped his soda.
   One EMT should perform the initial assessment and develop the history. He should speak slowly and clearly, be honest, and be supportive but decisive.
4. __ A middle-aged woman is upset that she is having breathing difficulties.
5. __ An elderly man is afraid that he will die if he enters a hospital.
6. X A young man threatens to kill all people who wear uniforms.
   Request police for safety. Have nonuniformed personnel approach the patient when it is safe to do so. One EMT should perform the initial assessment and develop the history. He should speak slowly and clearly, be honest, and be supportive but decisive.
7. __ A middle-aged man expresses anger that his wife just died.
8. __ A newly arrived immigrant cannot follow your directions.
9. __ A young man is upset after the saw he was using sliced his hand.
10. X A teenaged girl states she is going to stab all the snakes in the room.
    Request police for safety. Be sure the girl is unarmed. One EMT should perform the initial assessment and develop the history. He should speak slowly and clearly, be honest, and do not attempt to confirm or deny any hallucination..

True or False:

1. F	6. T
2. T	7. T
3. T	8. F
4. F	9. T
5. T	10. F

Short Answer:

1. They are assumed to not be in a frame of mind where they are capable of making decisions regarding their health.
2. Four people are recommended, in order to maintain the safety of the crew.
3. The EMT should sit at the head of the patient, where he can manage the ABCs and speak directly to the patient.
4. When a patient is restrained, pulses, movement, and sensation should be checked every 5–10 minutes.

Critical Thinking 1:

1. Yes, it is a situation in which the man's behavior is unacceptable to himself, family, or the community.
2. Yes, based on the medic alert bracelet, it is very probable that the behavior is being caused a malfunction of the brain due to incorrect sugar levels.
3. They should try to assist the man into the ambulance so that he is not being viewed by onlookers. They should call for ALS, as it is possible that the man will be unable to follow directions to take sugar, or that he will be unable to control his airway. They should request the police unit to try to contact the man's family.

Critical Thinking 2:

1. Yes, the patient is exhibiting behavior that is intolerable to self, family, or community.
2. The EMTs must be nonjudgmental and nonconfrontational, while ensuring they are able to withdraw as necessary. They should choose or alter their approach to avoid offending the patient.
3. Janie must remember that the patient is ill and comments made are under duress. She should not take the comments personally.

4. She should maintain a professional attitude, clearly identify herself, and state her intentions clearly.
5. Only one EMT should speak to the patient. This allows trust to be built and also decreases the possibilty of confusion.

Chapter 28

Matching:

1. i	6. k	11. d
2. l	7. m	12. j
3. o	8. b	13. e
4. a	9. c	14. g
5. h	10. n	15. f

Sorting:

	Radiation	Convection	Conduction	Evaporation
Removing your sweater in a cool room	X			
Sitting on cold rocks			X	
Breathing				X
Sitting in front of a fan		X		
Turning on the air conditioning in the house	X			
Entering a meat cooler	X			
Sweating				X
Swimming in a cold lake			X	
Standing in the wind		X		
Lying on a waterbed heated to 70° F			X	

Identification:

X	diabetes mellitus	__	sprained ankle
__	adolescent	X	thyroid condition
X	heart disease	X	head injury
X	multiple medications	X	shock
__	isolated broken wrist	__	infected tooth
X	generalized infection	X	spinal cord injury
X	burns		

Treatments:

Local cold injuries: remove patient from cold or wet environment, remove cold or wet clothing, rewarm injured part

Hypothermia: assess body temperature; remove patient from cold environment; remove cold, wet clothing; cover with warm blankets; administer oxygen (preferably warmed and humidified), prevent further heat loss

Heat cramps: remove patient from hot environment, gently massage painful area, rehydrate orally with water or electrolyte solution

Heat exhaustion: remove patient from hot environment, remove excess clothing, rehydrate orally with water or electrolyte solutions, call for ALS

Heat stroke: remove the patient from hot environment, provide aggressive cooling measures, monitor ABCs, administer oxygen, transport, call for ALS

Snakebites: keep patient calm, immobilize extremity, keep below level of heart, transport to hospital, consider ALS intercept

Sorting:

1.	X poor coordination	7.	X pale skin
2.	__ flushing	8.	__ stomach cramps
3.	__ nausea	9.	X mood changes
4.	X slurred speech	10.	X decreased sensation
5.	X poor judgment	11.	__ muscle cramps
6.	X slow pulse	12.	__ itching

Identification:

1.	active	3.	active
2.	passive	4.	passive

5.	passive	7.	active
6.	active	8.	passive

Ordering:

_3_	row	_4_	go
_1_	reach	_2_	throw

Listing:

descent: squeeze (air-filled spaces like sinus)

ascent: decompression sickness, pulmonary overpressurization, air embolism

Fill in the Blank:

Lightning strikes are divided into <u>MINOR</u> and <u>SEVERE</u> injuries. With lesser injuries, the common symptoms include <u>CON-FUSION</u>, <u>AMNESIA</u>, and short-term memory difficulties. A large percentage of people suffer ruptured <u>EARDRUMS</u>. They may also suffer <u>BLUNT</u> trauma. The EMT should <u>IMMOBILIZE</u> the patient to prevent any further injuries.

In other people, the electricity produces a shock that stops <u>CARDIAC</u> electrical activity and a full arrest occurs. Even if the heart resumes function, the <u>BRAIN</u> may continue to malfunction, preventing <u>RESPIRATORY</u> effort and resulting in hypoxia. The first priority in the management of a victim of a lightning strike is <u>SCENE SAFETY</u>.

Short Answer:

1. Any two: convection, conduction, radiation, or evaporation
2. Routine cellular metabolism and muscle contraction are internal ways for the body to gain heat. An external source is for the body to absorb heat from a warmer environment.
3. Vasoconstriction, piloerection
4. The old or very young may be unable to remove themselves from the environment, or put on or remove clothing. They have a variation in amount of insulation.
5. Afterdrop results from peripheral vasodilation resulting from application of warm items to the skin. The cold blood caught out in the periphery is then sent back to the core of the body, resulting in a temperature drop.
6. Neurological damage, respiratory difficulties.
7. Any injury resulting during a dive can leave the patient at risk for a drowning or near-drowning episode.
8. Mountain sickness results from a decreased amount of oxygen in the air. The patient has not acclimated to this decreased oxygen and therefore suffers symptoms of hypoxia. Oxygen is used to both treat the illness and assist in acclimating to the environment.

Critical Thinking 1:

1. Lightning strike
2. Scene safety
3. If the man on the ground is in cardiac arrest, they should care for him first.
4. Trauma, including spinal injuries due to falls

Critical Thinking 2:

1. They know that the event took place within the past 24 hours, as the mailman had noticed that she was fine yesterday.
2. They should provide general hypothermia management.

Critical Thinking 3:

1. He was likely bitten by a black widow spider.
2. Bandage the site of the bite and provide supportive care.
3. Yes, some black widow bites can result in death. George should receive a complete evaluation at the hospital.

Chapter 29

Matching:

1.	d	6.	h
2.	f	7.	i
3.	j	8.	b
4.	g	9.	c
5.	a	10.	e

Definitions:

1. allergic reaction: an expected activation of the immune system upon an exposure to a particular substance
2. epinephrine: an injectable medication that dilates the bronchioles and constricts the blood vessels
3. ingestion: taken in orally
4. inhalation: taken in through the respiratory tract
5. injected: taken in through a hole made in the skin
6. absorbed: taken in through intact skin
7. poisoning: exposure to a substance that results in illness

Identification:

1. injected
2. injected
3. ingested or absorbed
4. inhaled
5. inhaled
6. absorbed or inhaled
7. inhaled or absorbed
8. absorbed
9. ingested
10. inhaled

True or False:

1. T
2. F
3. F
4. F
5. T
6. T
7. F

Completion:

Generic name	activated charcoal
Trade name	Actidose, SuperChar
Indication	recent ingestion of susceptible poison
Contraindication	inability to control airway or swallow
Dose	1 gram/kg (50–100g adults)
Route	orally

Completion:

Generic Name	epinephrine
Trade name	EpiPen, Adrenalin
Indication	life-threatening allergic reaction
Contraindication	none as long as indicated
Dose	0.3–0.5 mg adults (contents of injector)
Route	intramuscular

Short Answer:

1. Mild = Localized swelling   Severe = More generalized swelling
2. Respiratory signs including throat tightness, shortness of breath, cough, wheezing, stridor, hoarseness, tachypnea
   Cardiovascular signs including tachycardia, hypotension, dizziness, hypoperfusion
   Sense of impending doom
   Decreasing mental status, increasing difficulty breathing, decreasing blood pressure

Critical Thinking 1:

1. Absorption through his hands.
2. He should lay down or sit down, wash or wipe the remainder of the paste off his skin, and be monitored by an EMT.

Critical Thinking 2:

1. Injected with fluid from the wasps.
2. She should be given high-flow oxygen, ALS should be called, and EpiPen administration could be considered if the indications for such are present.

Critical Thinking 3:

1. Inhalation of toxic gas
2. Once correctly trained personnel have removed Aimee from the apartment, she should be given high-flow oxygen, ventilated if necessary and ALS should be called.

Chapter 30

Matching:

1. g
2. h
3. j
4. a
5. f

6. b
7. d
8. i
9. e
10. c

Identification:

1. Battle's sign
2. Otorrhea
3. Raccoon eyes

4. Rhinorrhea
5. Cushing's triad

True or False:

1. F
2. T
3. F
4. T
5. T

6. F
7. T
8. T
9. T
10. F

Calculation:

1. 3/2/4 = 9
2. 4/5/6 = 15
3. 1/1/2 = 4

4. 1/1/1 = 3
5. 3/4/5 = 12

Sorting:

_X_ ventilate at up to 20 breaths per minute in the adult patient
_X_ elevate the head of the stretcher or board
___ stop CSF flow
_X_ control bleeding
___ determine exact diagnosis
___ withhold oxygen
_X_ provide rapid transport
___ avoid helicopter transport due to pressure changes
_X_ calculate GCS

Fill in the Blank:

The most important thing an EMT can do to improve the outcome of a head-injured patient is to adequately assess and manage the <u>AIRWAY</u>, <u>BREATHING</u>, and <u>CIRCULATORY</u> status. The brain needs adequate perfusion with well-<u>OXYGENATED</u> blood. After ensuring an adequate airway, assess the effectiveness of the patient's own <u>BREATHING</u>. Next, turn attention to the <u>CIRCULATORY</u> status.

For the patient who has suffered a significant injury, the EMT should then move on to a <u>RAPID</u> <u>TRAUMA</u> <u>ASSESSMENT</u>. For a high-priority patient, this will be done during transport. During both assessments completed up to this time, the <u>LEVEL</u> of <u>CONSCIOUSNESS</u>, or patient responsiveness, will be observed. This can be quantified on the <u>GLASGOW COMA</u> scale. A <u>TREND</u> or pattern that may be seen in repeated vital signs is an increased BP, decreased pulse rate, and changed respiratory pattern. This combination is called <u>CUSHING'S</u> <u>TRIAD</u>.

As with all high priority patients, be sure the patient is receiving high-<u>FLOW</u> <u>OXYGEN</u>. Ongoing assessments should be completed every 5 minutes.

Short Answer:

1. Swelling in the head makes it difficult for blood to flow to brain cells. An adequate or somewhat higher blood pressure is needed to overcome the swelling that has occurred. Hypotension in the head injured patient means that little to no blood will reach the brain cells.
2. The fontanelles are areas where the bones have not yet grown together and fused. Any swelling of brain tissue will seek an "escape" route and push through the open areas of the bones.

Critical Thinking 1:

1. Head, spine, and limb injuries are most likely.
2. They must provide C-spine stabilization, control the airway, provide oxygen and ventilate as necessary, and control any external bleeding.
3. AVPU and Glascow Coma Scale
4. They can elevate the head of the spine board slightly to facilitate venous drainage, and they can oxygenate/ventilate.

Critical Thinking 2:

1. They must provide C-spine stabilization, control the airway, provide oxygen, and ventilate as necessary. If there was any external bleeding, they would need to control that as well.
2. Decreasing mental status, persistent vomiting, a Glascow Coma Scale score of less than 8, unequal pupils, seizures, hypertension, bradycardia, changes in respiratory pattern
3. Surgical intervention

Chapter 31

Word Scramble:

1. paralysis
2. paraplegia
3. paresthesia
4. quadriplegia
5. priapism

Completion:

1. vertebrae
2. cervical
3. thoracic
4. lumbar
5. meninges

Fill in the Blank:

The first clue the EMT has as to the possibility of a spinal injury is the <u>MECHANISM</u> of <u>INJURY</u>. Knowing the stacked nature of the vertebrae will enable the EMT to imagine the injuries. In a motor vehicle collision, the most common injury type is <u>FLEXION/EXTENSION</u> of the neck. Falls can result in <u>BROKEN</u> bones that intrude into the cord, or <u>COMPRESSION</u> fractures that actually crush the vertebrae. The phenomenon, known as <u>AXIAL LOADING</u>, can cause trauma along the spinal column, especially in the lumbar region. Firearms can lead to spinal injuries due to the uncertainty of the <u>DIRECTION</u> of TRAVEL of the bullet. Sports injuries may also cause spinal injury.

True or False:

1. F
2. T
3. T
4. T
5. F
6. F
7. T
8. F
9. F
10. F

Short Answer:

1. The patient can suffer bone or ligament injuries that do not impinge on the cord. The patient should not be allowed to continue walking around, as these injuries make the column unstable and the cord suspectible to damage.
2. The patient has injured his coccyx. He has not sustained cord damage, however, as the cord ends at the second lumbar region.
3. The injury in the cervical region can impair messages from the respiratory center to the diaphragm.
4. There are no messages to the heart or blood vessels. This results in the heart not speeding up or the vessels redirectly flow away from the skin.
5. The EMT should try to avoid a head-tilt/chin-lift. Use a jaw thrust instead.

Critical Thinking:

1. Manual stabilization of spine; C-collar; short spinal device; to long spine board
2. Manual stabilization of spine; C-collar; rapid extrication to a long spine board
3. Manual stabilization of spine; C-collar; standing takedown to a long spine board

Chapter 32

Missing Letters:

cardiac contusion	hemothorax	flail segment
hemoptysis	abdomen	tension pneumothorax
eviseration	paradoxical motion	petechiae
sucking chest wound	pulmonary contusion	tracheal deviation
tamponade	subcutaneous emphysema	

Identification:

B	Subcutaneous emphysema	T	Jugular venous distension
B	Tachycardia	T	Loss of radial pulses
B	Tachypnea	T	Decreased lung compliance
B	Difficulty breathing	T	Hypotension
B	Diminished breath sounds	T	Tracheal deviation

Labeling: See Figure 32-1 in your text.

Completion:

1. blunt
2. bleeding
3. pain, breathing
4. DCAP-BTLS
5. subcutaneous emphysema
6. oxygenation, perfusion
7. hemothorax
8. occlusive dressing
9. three
10. affected

True or False:

1. T
2. T
3. F
4. F
5. F
6. F
7. F
8. T
9. T
10. T

Short Answer:

1. The treatment is the same. Trying to accurately diagnose takes time that could be better spent on speedy packaging. Recognition of abdominal trauma is the most important responsibility.
2. Covering with a moist sterile dressing offers protection from infection, saves the area from drying out, and conserves heat.

Critical Thinking:

1. They know he is alert, has an open airway at present, is breathing sufficiently well to enable him to yell, and his brain is sufficiently perfused to allow him to sit up and think through things.
2. While he was shot in the chest, it is a dynamic space. There is the potential for lung, rib, liver, and small intestine damage. Bone fragments from any shattered bone could also cause wider damage.
3. They should provide high-flow oxygen and closely monitor respirations. If necessary, be ready to ventilate. Cover the wound with an occlusive dressing. Call for ALS intercept if available.
4. Transport the patient on his affected side.
5. Open one side of the occlusive dressing. It is possible that covering the wound site allowed air to become trapped and pressure to be built up, creating a tension pneumothorax.

Chapter 33

Missing Letters:

contusion	incision	evisceration
amputation	impaled object	wound
hematoma	burns	lacerations
crush	avulsion	tattooing
abrasion	puncture	degloving

Identification:

1. cravat
2. bandage
3. gauze
4. triangle
5. dressing
6. trauma
7. pressure dressing
8. figure 8
9. occlusive
10. compress
11. recurrent dressing
12. roller bandage
13. spiral bandage
14. universal dressing
15. tourniquet

Definitions:

1. hemorrhage: a medical term for excessive bleeding
2. inflammation: the body's attempt to prevent infection and begin healing
3. necrotic: dead tissue
4. coagulation: the process of blood clotting
5. ecchymosis: a wider collection of blood under the skin caused by a rupture of a large blood vessel
6. embolism: a physical blockage in the bloodstream
7. fasciotomy: a surgical procedure whereby the skin is cut to relieve pressure

True or False:

1. T
2. F
3. F
4. F
5. F
6. T
7. T
8. F

Sorting:

Arterial bleeding	Venous bleeding	Capillary bleeding
spurting	constant	watery
pulsing	deep red	seeping
bright red	pouring out of wound	oozing
	rivulets	

Calculation:

1. 18%
2. 27%
3. 28%
4. 1–1.5%
5. 18%
6. 1%
7. 18%
8. 31.5%
9. 1%
10. 4.5%

Identification:

1. superficial
2. superficial
3. full thickness
4. partial thickness
5. full thickness
6. full thickness
7. full thickness
8. full thickness
9. partial thickness
10. superficial

Short Answer:

1. Blistering opens the skin, permitting germs to enter. Also, the patient was around equipment that may have been unclean.
2. There is no way to determine the exact trajectory of the bullet. Additionally, other injuries that may have occurred in conjunction with the GSW may lead to patient decompensation.
3. The object may be preventing a loss of blood. Removing it would allow the blood to flow freely.
4. Bleeding from the cheek can be controlled from both outside and inside the mouth. It is difficult to control the airway with an object impaled into the cheek.

Critical Thinking 1:

1. Airway and bleeding
2. Airway management, high-flow oxygen, occlusive dressing to the wound, bleeding control
3. Mark remains at risk for an air embolism, which would interfere with blood flow and could lead to hypoxia.

Critical Thinking 2:

1. A sucking chest wound
2. Respiratory distress
3. Airway management, high-flow oxygen, ventilate as needed, occlusive dressing to the chest wound, bleeding control

Chapter 34

Identification:
1. Humerus, radius, ulna
2. Carpals, metacarpals, and phalanges
3. Femur, patella, tibia, and fibula
4. Tarsals, matatarsals, calcaneus, phalanges
5. Scapula, clavicles, ribs, sternum, vertebrae, pelvis

Definitions:
1. closed fracture: a broken bone in which the bone ends do not break the skin
2. dislocation: a bone that slips out of the joint, out of alignment
3. dorsiflexion: movement of the toes upward toward the nose
4. footdrop: a loss of nervous control that results in a flaccid foot
5. locked: a bone that is unable to return to its natural position
6. motor nerves: the nervous tissue that carries messages to initiate muscular contraction
7. open fracture: a broken bone in which the bone ends erupt through the skin
8. osteoporosis: a softening of bones due to loss of calcium
9. position of function: the natural relaxed position of the hand or foot
10. range of motion: the movement of bone or limb allowed by a joint
11. sciatic nerve: the primary sensory and motor nerve of the legs
12. sensory nerve: the nervous tissue that carries impulses of feeling such as pressure or pain
13. spontaneous reduction: a bone that returns to its natural position without assistance
14. sprain: a stretch of a ligament or tendon beyond its range of motion resulting in tissue injury.
15. traction: a steady inline pull

Matching:
1. f
2. g
3. a
4. c
5. b
6. e
7. d

True or False:
1. F
2. T
3. F
4. T
5. F
6. F
7. T
8. T
9. T
10. T
11. T
12. F
13. T
14. F
15. T

Fill in the Blank:
Next to most <u>LONG BONES</u> lies an artery, a <u>NERVE</u>, and a <u>VEIN</u>. Surrounding the bone are muscles, <u>TENDONS</u>, and soft tissues. Covering all of this is skin. If a broken bone end cuts an artery, there will be bleeding into the tissues, causing the area to become <u>PAINFUL</u>, <u>SWOLLEN</u>, and <u>DEFORMED</u>. Disruption of an artery can cause loss of <u>PULSES</u> distal to the injury.

If a sensory nerve is injured, the patient may complain of numbness or tingling, called <u>PARESTHESIA</u>. If the motor nerve has been injured, however, the EMT may see signs of weakness of movement or <u>PARESIS</u>. If there is no movement of the extremity or <u>PARALYSIS</u>, check the opposite extremity. Loss of movement on both sides should alert the EMT to possible <u>SPINAL</u> injury.

A grating sensation called <u>CREPITUS</u> can often be noted when the patient moves an injured extremity. This is caused by bone ends <u>GRINDING</u> against each other. It is not necessary for the EMT to elicit this! Sudden pain at the exact location of the injury is called <u>POINT TENDERNESS</u>.

During the general impression, the EMT may notice that the patient is protecting or self-splinting an injury. This is called <u>GUARDING</u>.

Listing:
1. Swelling
2. Pain
3. Deformity
4. Paralysis
5. Paresthesia
6. Pulselessness
7. Cyanosis
8. Crepitus
9. Point tenderness
10. Guarding/self-splinting

Reviewing:
1. Deformity
2. Contusion
3. Abrasion
4. Puncture
5. Burns
6. Tenderness
7. Laceration
8. Swelling

Short Answer:
1. Movement of the joints can cause movement of the bone ends, leading to pain and soft tissue damage.
2. Adjacent to the joints is an artery and a nerve. Attempting to realign the joint can cause them to become trapped, leading to further injury distal to the joint.
3. It may be impossible or impractical to transport the patient out of the wilderness. Because hospitals are closer in urban areas, this is unnecessary in most cases.

Critical Thinking 1:
1. Michael is awake, has an open airway, is breathing, and has adequate circulation at the moment. They know his arm hurts and he is self-splinting it.
2. Scene survey, general first impression, initial assessment, focused history, physical
3. Manually stabilize the arm. Check pulses, movement, and sensation. Apply a rigid splint padding any voids. Keep the hand in a position of function. Secure the splint. Recheck pulses, movement, and sensation. Place the arm in a sling. Elevate it. Apply ice.
4. Yes, they would need to cover it with a dry, sterile dressing and splint in position found.
5. One attempt may be made to realign the ends and restore pulses. Consider contacting Medical Control.

Critical Thinking 2:
1. Most likely a patella dislocation
2. Agree

Chapter 35

True or False:
1. F
2. T
3. F
4. F
5. F
6. T
7. F
8. T
9. T
10. T

Identification:
1. Abortion
2. Eclampsia
3. Placenta previa
4. Supine hypotensive syndrome
5. Appendicitis
6. Miscarriage
7. Ectopic pregnancy
8. Placental abruption

Fill in the Blank:

Pregnancy changes the way the body takes care of itself. The pregnant woman's heart is normally <u>HIGHER</u> than the nonpregnant woman, and her blood pressure is usually <u>LOWER</u>. The EMT should remember that the pregnant woman has manufactured approximately <u>30</u>% more blood than usual, and so a significant blood loss can occur before there is a change in <u>VITAL SIGNS</u>.

The EMT must remember that in managing any trauma in pregnancy, he must concentrate on saving the <u>MOTHER</u>.

Short Answer:
1. Skin signs; the normal vital signs have been changed by the process of pregnancy. The mother in shock will shunt blood away from the fetus and also away from the skin. The EMT can make observations about the skin.
2. Falls, blunt trauma in MVC, intentional violence
3. The mother's center of gravity changes, placing her at greater risk of losing her balance. In MVC, the abdomen is likely to strike the steering wheel or dash first. Pregnancy causes many emotions, not only in the woman but also her partner, placing her at risk for domestic violence.

Critical Thinking:

1. Scene safety/size-up, general first impression, initial assessment, focused history and physical, vital signs. Pay attention to the skin signs.
2. Placenta previa
3. They should manage her in the same way regardless of the cause. Place her supine and turned to her left side. Give high-flow oxygen. Call for ALS if not done already. Transport to an appropriate facility. Continue with ongoing assessments.

Chapter 36

Word Scramble:

1. effacement
2. labor
3. multiparous
4. primiparous
5. crowning
6. gravida
7. para
8. molding
9. meconium

Definitions:

1. amniotic sac: the membranous sac that surrounds the fetus in the uterus
2. cervical dilation: progressive opening of the cervix that occurs as the fetal head descends into the pelvis
3. bloody show: expulsion of a small amount of bloody mucous from the cervix as it begins to thin
4. Braxton Hicks contractions: random contractions that occur in the third trimester; also known as false labor
5. cardinal movements of labor: series of natural movements the infant makes upon descent through the birth canal
6. prolapsed umbilical cord: presentation of the umbilical cord before the infant; results in compression of the cord
7. breach presentation: presentation of foot or buttocks first instead of the infant's head
8. premature delivery: a delivery that occurs before the 37th week of the pregnancy

Sorting:

First stage	Second stage	Third stage
effacement	delivery of the infant	delivery of the placenta
rupture of amniotic sac	infant's head pushing on rectum	gushing of blood
full cervical dilation	crowning	about 250–500 cc

Identification:

1. X Due date
2. ___ Blood pressure
3. X Any complications during the pregnancy
4. ___ Crowning
5. X Prenatal care
6. ___ Any fluids from the vagina
7. X Time when contractions started
8. ___ BSI
9. ___ Maternal weight
10. X How long each contraction lasts
11. X Gravida
12. X Parity

Sorting:

Field delivery	Transport
crowning	primiparous, contractions 10 minutes apart
multiparous, contractions 2 minutes apart	irregular contractions
need to move bowels	primiparous, regular contractions, no observation of fetal head
need to push	
increased vaginal pressure	

Listing:

1. Surgical scissors are used to cut the cord.
2. Clamps are used to clamp the cord in two places.
3. Bulb syringe is used to suction the mouth and nose.
4. Towels are used to dry the infant.
5. Gauze sponges are used to wipe blood.
6. BSI is necessary for self-protection. There are many fluids during a delivery.
7. The blanket is to keep the infant warm.
8. A plastic bag is used to transport the placenta to the hospital.

Ordering:

_9_	Deliver placenta	_1_	BSI
_2_	Position the mother	_7_	Clamp cord when pulsations have stopped
_3_	Gentle pressure on the infant's head during crowning	_8_	Dry infant and wrap
_4_	Check for cord around the neck	_6_	Support the infant's weight during delivery
_10_	Record time and place of delivery	_11_	Transport mother, infant, and placenta to hospital
_5_	Suction mouth and then nose of infant		

Critical Thinking:

1. See Table 36-2 in your text.
2. The EMTs need to tell Grace that delivery is imminent, and that they will assist her in delivering her infant at home. They need to be supportive.
3. Yes, since Grace has not had prenatal care and her infant is arriving early (premature), the EMTs would be wise to obtain any needed advice.
4. Twins
5. The EMTs need to prepare for the second delivery by obtaining a second OB kit and by calling for additional personnel.

Chapter 37

True or False:

1. F
2. T
3. F
4. F
5. F
6. T
7. F
8. F
9. F
10. T

Sorting:

___ suckling
_X_ placing the newborn on a table (place on a blanket or towel)
___ positioning the newborn on mother's abdomen
_X_ leaving baby's head uncovered to monitor fontanelles (dry and cover the head)
_X_ letting infant stay in amniotic fluid (dry the infant)
swaddling

Ordering:

_5_	ALS drugs	_1_	Drying, warming, and positioning
_2_	Blow-by oxygen	_3_	BVM
_4_	Chest compressions		

Fill in the Blank:

Measuring heart rate, respiratory effort, muscle tone, responses, and color in the newborn is determined through the use of the APGAR score. It is completed at 1 and 5 minutes after birth. The EMT must also assess the newborn's airway. Place the newborn supine and slightly head down. Use a BULB SYRINGE to clear the infant's NOSTRILS. The newborn is an obligate NOSE breather. Respirations must be adequate. Crying is a good sign. Even though respirations are adequate, the infant may have blue hands and feet. This is called ACROCYANOSIS. A heart rate of less than 60 beats per minute means that the EMT must begin chest compressions. Once the initial assessment and APGAR is completed, begin a FOCUSED medical assessment. Sometimes the infant's head may appear misshapen. This results from the birth and is called MOLDING. The head shape will return to normal. The EMT must assess the UMBILICAL cord, which should appear bluish white. The EMT must take care to appear professional and nonjudgmental, as new parents "read" the expressions and behaviors of the caregivers.

Calculation:

1. 9
2. 2
3. 7
4. 1
5. 10

Short Answer:

1. The infant produces a lot of mucous during its first few minutes to hours, and the infant is an obligate nose breather.
2. Nasal flaring, bradycardia, retractions, seesaw respirations, grunting

Critical Thinking:

1. 1
2. ABCs, utilizing the inverted pyramid of newborn care
3. Honesty, complete explanation of all care

Chapter 38

Word Scramble:

1. croup
2. asthma
3. meningitis
4. epiglottitis
5. debriefing
6. retractions
7. febrile

Completion:

See Table 38-1 of your text.

True or False:

1.	T	6.	T	11.	T
2.	F	7.	T	12.	F
3.	F	8.	F	13.	F
4.	T	9.	T	14.	T
5.	T	10.	F	15.	T

Matching:

1.	i	6.	c
2.	h	7.	d
3.	f	8.	j
4.	g	9.	e
5.	b	10.	a

Correcting:

1. Unknown
2. 1 week and 1 year
3. Sleeping
4. Lower
5. Remove the word NOT
6. Cannot
7. During the resuscitation
8. Remove the word NOT

Short Answer:

1. Aspiration of a foreign body
2. The child's airway is smaller and more likely to become obstructed by swelling.
3. No, the two illnesses are treated the same way in the field.
4. Signs of hypoperfusion include: increased heart rate, pale skin color, delayed capillary refill, nausea, a decreased urinary output, changes in the child's level of consciousness, and an eventual drop in blood pressure.

Critical Thinking 1:

1. Yes, there are signs that this child has a severe illness called meningitis.
2. The EMTs should wear gloves and a mask.
3. The EMTs need to provide explanations of what they are doing, and give caring support to Mrs. Smythe.

Critical Thinking 2:

1. No
2. The child has a good airway, as evidenced by his cough and yelling.

Chapter 39

Fill in the Blank:

1. mandated reporter
2. mechanical ventilator
3. cerebrospinal fluid shunt
4. tracheostomy

5. child abuse
6. feeding tube

7. tracheostomy tube
8. central venous catheter

Identification:

Toddlers	motor vehicle collisions
	pools and buckets
	scalding
	household cleaners/pills
School-age	motor vehicle collisions
	bikes
	intentional fires
Adolescents	motor vehicle collisions
	suicide/homicide
	drug ingestion/overdose

Assessments:

General impression: Compare this child's actions to those of a noninjured child. Any answers indicating a deviation from age norms are acceptable.

Mental status: inactive, lack of attention to environment, dull eyes, self-absorbed

Airway: breathing through open mouth (air hunger)

Breathing: seesaw respirations, retractions

Circulation: pale, cool, tachycardic, delayed capillary refill

Short Answer:

1. A child's head is larger, proportionally. This makes him more top heavy and more prone to head injuries.
2. Comfort and cooperation from a child in more familiar surroundings, or convenience of move from vehicle to ambulance
3. Swelling in the airway, inhalations of toxins from the fire, hypothermia
4. Pattern of injury does not match reported mechanism of injury, several injuries in various stages of healing, responding to same address repeatedly for injuries. The EMT should document accurately and without making judgments. The EMT should also report his observations to the physician.
5. Children with special needs may have vital signs and responses that are not usual for most children but are normal for that child. Caregivers usually have a clear understanding of baseline information.

Identification:

1. trauma center
2. local hospital
3. local hospital
4. trauma center
5. trauma center

6. trauma center
7. trauma center
8. trauma center
9. local hospital
10. trauma center

Chapter 40

Matching:

1. i
2. a
3. g
4. j
5. b

6. h
7. c
8. f
9. d
10. e

Identification:

1. Visual acuity declines
2. Progressive decline in hearing
3. Stiffening of blood vessels
   Build up of fatty deposits in blood vessels
   Decrease in exercise tolerance
   Diminished effectiveness of heart as a pump

4. Decreased elasticity of chest wall and lung tissue, indicating a decrease in lung volume
   Inefficiency of cilia and cough mechanism
   Decreased oxygen uptake
5. Loss of teeth
   Decreased motility of GI tract, with inefficient absorption of nutrients
6. Decline in kidney function
   Loss of bladder tone and capacity
7. Loss of calcium from bone
   Decreased flexibility in joints
8. Loss of fat beneath the skin
   Decreased effectiveness of sweat glands

Fill in the Blank:

In the elderly, a <u>HEART</u> attack may present itself atypically, without the classic complaint of chest pain. This is called a silent <u>MYOCARDIAL</u> <u>INFARCTION</u>.

While a stroke or <u>CEREBROVASCULAR</u> accident can occur at any age, it is more likely to occur in the elderly. The neurological changes that occur result from a disruption of <u>BLOOD</u> <u>FLOW</u> to brain tissue. Because the damage is <u>IRRE-VERSIBLE</u>, the person will lose a part of his body function. The most common type of stroke is an <u>ISCHEMIC</u> stroke resulting from a blockage of blood flow. The other type of stroke results from bleeding into brain tissue and is called a <u>HEMORRHAGIC</u> stroke. The most common type of stroke results in damage to an area that allows movement of arms, legs, and face. Therefore, symptoms of a stroke include <u>WEAKNESS</u> of the arms and legs, and <u>DIFFICULTY</u> speaking.

Listing:

1. Mental status
2. Pupil exam
3. Pronator drift
4. Facial droop
5. Clarity of speech

Short Answer:

1. Level of consciousness declines in delirium; it remains normal in dementia.
2. Delirium is usually caused by an acute medical condition that can be treated and reversed.

Critical Thinking:

1. Dementia, likely Alzheimer's disease
2. They must consider vascular problems, subdural hemorrhage or other trauma, infections, alcohol use or drug intoxication, and depression.
3. No, patients with Alzheimer's disease may develop a worsening of their symptoms when other medical conditions are present.
4. Lisa and Tony should perform a complete patient assessment, including initial assessment, focused history, and physical, as well as obtain a complete history from the son. It may be advisable to obtain information from the Adult Day Service Center also.
5. The son needs emotional support; it is often difficult to provide care for elderly parents. He also needs a step-by-step explanation of the reasons for the exam and history gathering.
6. Optimal care would include placing the woman on the stretcher in a comfortable position, obtaining a complete set of vital signs, respectfully obtaining the physical exam, and transporting the woman to a hospital. Of key importance is respect and compassion for the woman and her family.

Chapter 41

Definitions:

1. A method to make a patient's wishes about resuscitation known to family and health care providers
2. A physician's order to not start CPR or revive a patient in cardiac arrest
3. A person chosen to make medical decisions on behalf of another
4. Legal documents directing a patient's care if he becomes unable to do so
5. A designated person to make decisions for another

True or False:

1.	F	6.	F
2.	F	7.	F
3.	T	8.	T
4.	T	9.	T
5.	T	10.	T

Short Answer:
1. Consent and the right to withhold consent
2. The first two are legal documents requiring attorney involvement, while the second two require physician involvement.

Critical Thinking 1:
1. The EMTs need to assess the patient and determine if she is apneic and pulseless. If their system allows acceptance of a DNR, then they should honor the DNR. If they cannot honor it, they must give clear explanation to the family. Any questions can be directed to the Medical Control physician.
2. Regardless of the outcome, the granddaughter needs support and the opportunity to express her grief.

Critical Thinking 2:
1. Based on the unclear situation, the EMTs should begin resuscitation under the doctrine of implied consent. Questions can be directed to the Medical Control physician.

Chapter 42

Matching:

1.	k	6	n	11.	e
2.	h	7.	b	12.	o
3.	f	8.	m	13.	g
4.	l	9.	d	14.	j
5.	a	10.	c	15.	i

Definitions:
1. controlled intersection: an intersection with a traffic control device
2. yelp: a sharp, quick chirping type siren sound
3. LZ officer: designated person at scene of an incident who is responsible for choosing a landing zone and ensuring its safety
4. covering the brake: placing one foot over the brake in anticipation of stopping
5. surrounding area: space above and around the helicopter touchdown site
6. emergency ambulances: vehicles specifically designed for patient transportation
7. four-second rule: the amount of time separating the emergency vehicle from the one in front of it; usually calculated against a fixed object such as a pole or parked car.
8. emergency services vehicle: a vehicle used by either fire, police, or EMS department
9. touchdown area: area within the landing zone where helicopter will actually land
10. wail: a steady siren sound that ascends and then descends in pitch

Listing:
1. trained
2. rested
3. physically prepared
4. mentally prepared

Listing:
1. required items are where they belong
2. items function
3. electrical equipment is charged
4. batteries are charged
5. oxygen is available, portable tanks are filled and functional
6. equipment is clean

Listing:
See Table 42-5 in your text.

Listing:
See Table 42-5 in your text.

Descriptions:

1. Alarm and alert: communications center notified of event; may EMD[QA] the call
2. Initial information: communication specialist will give EMT sufficient information to find the call, know what equipment might be necessary, and be aware of any special concerns such as access
3. Departure: locate call on map, disconnect shoreline, crew members wear seat belts
4. Driving: using appropriate response mode, red lights and sirens for high priority, normal speed and following all traffic laws for low priority
5. Arrival: position ambulance, notify communications
6. On-scene actions: keep communications aware; nature of incident, number of patients, added resources, patient assessment and care, packaging and movement of patient to ambulance
7. Transport to facility: decision as to how and what priority, secure patient and crew in vehicle
8. Arrival at facility: notify communications, position ambulance
9. Transfer of care: move patient from ambulance cot to facility stretcher, raise siderails, lock wheels, secure equipment such as IV lines or oxygen, give complete verbal report, give patient belongings to receiving staff, provide written documentation
10. Preparation for next call: clean, decontaminate and restock, ensure adequate fuel

Critical Thinking:

1. Based on mechanism of injury, extent of injury, and a lengthy extrication; the helicopter appears to be a good choice for transport.
2. Choose a landing zone as close to scene as is safely possible

   Have a space of 75–100 square feet

   Have a slope of less than 10 degrees

   Surrounding area free of obstacles

   Mark the landing zone

   Observe the descent of the helicopter. Wave pilot off if landing becomes unsafe

   Remain in sight of the pilot. Do not permit anyone to approach until signaled by the pilot. Approach should be from the front at 12 o'clock position.

Chapter 43

Definitions:

1. chain of command: a system where every person has a superior, and that superior then reports to the Incident Commander
2. command post: area where fire, EMS, and police run a unified command of the incident
3. decontamination corridor: area that bridges the hot and cold zones; hazardous materials are cleaned off personnel here
4. hot zone: immediate area of a HAZMAT spill; obvious risk to personnel at this area
5. material safety data sheets (MSDS): listing of health and safety information on various substances
6. multiple casualty incident (MCI): an event where the number of patients outweigh the number of EMTs
7. NFPA 704 symbol: a diamond-shaped warning sign, with four or more smaller diamonds inside of the larger one
8. START triage system: a popular triage system, standing for "Simple Triage And Rapid Treatment"
9. placard: system of symbols, indicating a certain class of hazardous material
10. triage: prioritizing patients based upon urgency

Matching:

1. c
2. f
3. i
4. e
5. g
6. j
7. h
8. d
9. b
10. a

Listing:

1. yellow
2. green
3. red
4. green
5. yellow
6. black
7. red
8. red
9. yellow
10. black

Ordering:

6	Warm zone is established with a decontamination corridor	8	Patients are decontaminated
5	Hot zone is established	9	Patients are treated
4	HAZMAT team is dispatched	2	EMS command is established
1	The first unit arrives at the scene of a rolled over tanker truck	10	Patients are transported
7	Patients are extracted from the tanker	3	Ambulance is staged in the cold zone

Research:

1. camphor
2. gasoline
3. helium
4. potassium cyanide
5. propyl alcohol, normal

6. 1415
7. 1514
8. 1692
9. 1072
10. 2802
11. Move victim to fresh air
   Call 911
   Apply artificial respiration if not breathing. DO NOT use mouth to mouth if victim has ingested the substance
   Administer oxygen
   Remove and isolate clothing
   Flush skin or eyes for 20 minutes
   Avoid spreading material
   Keep victim quiet and warm
   Note effects may be delayed
   Ensure all medical personnel are aware of the substance involved and take steps to protect self

Critical Thinking 1:

1. Establish command and designate a command post
   Declare an emergency and implement any preplans
   Appoint officers
   Coordinate with other emergency agencies
   Relinquish command when appropriately relieved
2. Safety officer, staging, triage, treatment, and transportation
3. Appoint a Public Information Officer

Critical Thinking 2:

1. *North American Emergency Response Guidebook* by placard
   CHEMTREC
   Shipping papers
   (less specific) placard symbols and colors
2. Call for resources and establish a perimeter
3. Hot zone: special units
   Cold zone: EMS and other emergency workers

Chapter 44

Matching:

1.	f	6.	a
2.	d	7.	b
3.	g	8.	e
4.	i	9.	j
5.	h	10.	c

Identification:

1.	V	3.	V
2.	V	4.	V

5. W   8. W
6. W   9. W
7. V   10. B

Identification:
1. Personal protective equipment   5. Safety vest
2. Ear plugs   6. Turnout coat
3. Boots and gloves   7. Helmet
4. Goggles

Short Answer:
1. Swift water:
   EMS plays primarily a supporting role!
   Locate the victim
   Attempt a shore-based rescue (reach, throw), if realistic
   Establish a base for the dive team
   Always wear a PFD if you are near the water
   Flat water:
   Reach
   Throw
   Row
   Then go if no other alternative means of rescue is avaliable
   Always wear a PFD
2. Phases of a rescue include: command, size-up, access and rescue, treatment, and transport
3. Helmet, eye protection, rip-resistant coat, heavy-duty work gloves

Critical Thinking 1:
1. Heavy rescue
2. Any three might include traffic, unstable tractor with load of sand, cab over bridge

Critical Thinking 2:
1. Shore rescue
2. Any three might include water itself, debris in the water, fuel in the water

Critical Thinking 3:
1. Confined space
2. Any three might include uneven terrain; falling rocks; lack of lighting, water, cool temperatures

Chapter 45

Definitions:
1. laryngoscope: tool used to visualize the glottic opening
2. hyperventilation: faster-than-normal rate of ventilation
3. cricoid pressure: partially occludes the esophagus, reducing the amount of air placed into the stomach during ventilation
4. 12-lead ECG: a collection of twelve different views of the heart's electrical activity
5. normal saline (NS): the most common IV fluid; consisting of salt and water
6. D5W: 5% dextrose in water; consisting of sugar and water
7. macrodrip: allows for rapid administration of fluid
8. lactated Ringer's solution: used in same situations as NS; it is an electrolyte fluid
9. microdrip: used for delivering less fluid to a patient
10. preoxygenation: oxygen is delivered to the patient prior to intubation

Ordering:
1   Check the solution for clarity and date.
3   Remove the tab from the solution, and the cap from the drip chamber.
2   Select IV tubing size, open the packaging, and close the roller clamp.
6   Open the roller clamp and allow the fluid through the IV tubing.

<u>4</u>   Put the tubing spike into the appropriate IV solution port on the IV bag.

<u>5</u>   Hold the solution upright, and squeeze the chamber to fill the drip chamber halfway with fluid.

Short Answer:

1. Key "Do Nots"
   Do not recap a needle
   Do not stick a needle into a seat or mattress
   Do not throw a needle
   Do not throw away sharps in anything but an approved container

2. Ways in which an EMT can help an ALS provider to intubate:
   Apply cricoid pressure, allowing the vocal chords to come into view more easily, also reducing the amount of air being pushed into the stomach
   Preoxygenate the patient, prior to the arrival of ALS
   Provide suctioning of the airway, so that the ALS provider can see the chords
   Secure the endotracheal tube (ETT) after intubation
   Confirm ETT placement by listening to lungs and epigastric sounds
   Hyperventilate the patient for 30 seconds just prior to an intubation attempt

3. Right arm
   Left arm
   Right leg
   Left leg

V^1: 4th right intercostal space at sternal border
V^2: 4th left intercostal space at sternal border
V^3: between V^2 and V^4
V^4: 5th left intercostal space midclavicle line
V^5: 5th left intercostal space anterior axillary line
V^6: 5th left intercostal space midaxillary line

See Figure 45-7 in your text.